White Coat Tales

White Coat Tales

Medicine's Heroes, Heritage, and Misadventures

Robert B. Taylor, MD

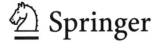 Springer

Robert B. Taylor, MD
Department of Family Medicine
School of Medicine
Oregon Health & Sciences University
Portland, OR 97239
USA

Library of Congress Control Number: 2007928818

ISBN: 978-0-387-73079-0   e-ISBN: 978-0-387-73080-6

Printed on acid-free paper.

9 8 7 6 5 4 3 2 1

springer.com

This book is dedicated to my family:
Anita, who has lovingly, but critically, reviewed
every page I ever wrote,

and

Our daughters, Diana and Sharon, who have
patiently listened to my stories over the years and
who have always supported my writing,

and

Our grandchildren, Francesca, Elizabeth, Jack,
and Annie, who are our hope for the future, and
who always make us proud.

Preface

If you want to understand today, you have to search yesterday.

Pearl S. Buck (1892–1973)

I begin this book with a premise: If there is a human endeavor that is richer in tradition, culture, and idiosyncrasies than medicine, I don't know what it is. What you are about to read presents some of these treasures—tales of the epic scientific discoveries as well as some behind-the-scenes medical anecdotes. In the pages that follow, you will find a selection of medicine's scientific triumphs, clinical curiosities, insightful aphorisms, inventive mnemonics, imaginative myths, and occasional blunders. In short, the book tells what physicians didn't learn in medical school, but probably should have. But the book is not intended solely for physicians. The tales that follow should be enlightening for all involved in medicine, including the diverse panorama of health professionals, and also anyone who has ever been a patient in a doctor's office or hospital.

What is different about this book that sets it apart from other books about medical history, lists of word origins, catalogs of clinical errors, and the like? First of all, the various items in this book—such as the probability that surgeon John Hunter (1728–1793) accidentally inoculated himself with syphilis as part of an experiment—"His autoinoculation seems to have confused gonorrhea with syphilis . . ." (1)—or the acronym to remember the muscles of mastication (it's BITEM)—are discussed in the context of themes rather than as alphabetical lists. Themes found in various chapters include the heroic traits and personal foibles of the giants of medical history, diseases and syndromes with historic footnotes, retrospective diagnoses of famous persons in history, and some medical trivia that helps humanize our heritage.

Secondly, the book is intended to be a primer, and I have not sought to be exhaustively comprehensive. Instead, the book describes a selection of what I consider to be noteworthy and intriguing items. As examples, modern cancer chemotherapy can trace its origins to the battlefields of World War

I (2), and the burial place of physician-scholar Moses Maimonides was determined in 1204 when his body was placed on a donkey that was then allowed to wander freely in Galilee (3). In the 19th century, Joseph Lister had no hand in formulating Listerine, but he did have an opinion about the product. By presenting only what I consider the most fascinating items, I am spared the quest for completeness that can make a book both ho-hum and far too long.

The book is reflective, and as the sole author, I share some personal insights. These include instances when various items were significant in medical training and clinical practice, including when I first learned a clinical concept or an aphorism that later helped make a difficult diagnosis, or when a tidbit of medical lore has led me to search out a fact that, perhaps, made me a better doctor, in both the healer and teacher sense of the word.

This book was fun to write; it should be read for pleasure. But because we physicians always need to be doing something "useful," the reader may also learn some things that are clinically helpful. For example, should we patch a corneal abrasion? Can the patient with congestive heart failure safely receive beta-blockers? What is the serotonin syndrome and why should physicians know about it? You will find the answers in this book. Inevitably, a few intrepid souls will want to dig deeper; for them, I have listed the sources used to locate and confirm entries in the text.

The key persons who assisted with this book were my wife and colleague, Anita D. Taylor, M.A.Ed., who offered numerous useful suggestions, and Coelleda O'Neil, who helped in many phases of manuscript preparation.

For me, preparing this volume has afforded countless happy hours rummaging about reference sources trying to find, for example, who first said, "When you hear hoofbeats, look for horses, not zebras," and the 14th century logical principle that this aphorism reprises. (See chapter 7 on Medical Aphorisms.) And why did the medieval epidemic of gangrene come to be called St. Anthony's fire and how is this historical entity related to medical practice today? (See chapter 4 on Medical Words and Phrases.) In fact, I have been collecting items for this book for three decades, and now—in semi-retirement—I have the chance to bring them together and share them with you.

For you, the reader, perhaps this book will prove to be only the beginning, and reading the pages that follow will prompt you to continue your study. Pick up a book in the reading list, search a medical connection in history on the Internet, learn the origin of a newly encountered medical word, or track an aphorism to its source. In short, I urge you to expand your horizons by learning more about medicine's heroes, heritage, and misadventures— the *White Coat Tales* that we all share.

Robert B. Taylor, MD
Portland, Oregon

References

1. Garrison FH. *A History of Medicine*, 4th ed. Philadelphia, PA: Saunders; 1929:347.
2. Cancer Research UK Web site. Available at: http://www.cancerresearchuk.org. Accessed May 21, 2007.
3. Rosner F. *The Medical Legacy of Moses Maimonides*. Hoboken, NJ: KTAV Publishing; 1998.

Contents

About This Book

The story of medicine is a tale of superstition and mysticism, empiricism and experimentation, heroism and entrepreneurism. The players are doctors and scientists, patients and families, victors and survivors involved in a variety of medical adventures. The plot involves instances of keen observation, dazzling insights, and fortuitous discoveries, such as when in 1920, a medical student noted that patients given mercury injections to treat syphilis passed large quantities of urine, suggesting that mercurials might have useful diuretic properties.

This work began as a study of medical word origins—our legacy from ancient Greek, Latin, Arabic, and a dozen other tongues. This promised to be a very straightforward task. But things change once you begin a journey, and I found myself wandering down dozens of beguiling side paths. The stories of medical words took me to mythology, wry quotations, assorted illnesses of famous persons, great deeds in medicine, and a few missteps on the perilous road to optimum health care. Thus, this is not an etymologic dictionary, nor is it your typical scholarly chronicle of medical history. In fact, the book contains a lot of stories not found in traditional medical history books (and, yes, some of those stories are found elsewhere but perhaps are told here with a new twist).

As I did research for the book, I came to think of it as an "archeological dig." As I excavated deeper into the stories of physicians, diseases, and medical scholarship, I discovered "shards" of interesting facts. These included how the Beatles—yes, John, Paul, George, and Ringo—played a role in the development of the computed tomography (CT) scanner. And how Winston Churchill termed his recurrent bouts of depression, "my black dog."

Fundamentally, this is a book about threads, connections, and the rich fabric of medical thinking. I tell about the how the admonition to "do no harm" evolved from a Hindu physicians' oath to influence Hippocrates, Thomas Sydenham, Florence Nightingale, and eventually a popular television show about a rural family physician. I describe how typhus and a fierce winter combined to defeat Napoleon in Russia. And I include some slip-ups, such as why there was a decade-plus lag between Alexander Fleming's 1928 discovery that *Penicillium* mold inhibited bacterial growth and the clinical use of penicillin, and why George Washington's death in 1799 may have been due more to the robust bleeding therapy employed by his physicians than to his throat infection. In the end, I hope that you have a richer understanding of medicine—our most noble profession.

I have tried not to just present an aphorism, acrostic, or anecdote without some background. For example, "All that wheezes is not asthma" makes more sense when placed in some historical or clinical context. Whenever possible, I have included a bit of a story about the book's entries.

The astute reader will soon note that among the physicians, scientists, and others mentioned in this book, most are men. This fact does not indicate some latent misogynous sentiment on my part; the historical fact is that since the days of early well-intentioned gourd rattling, the advances and pithy quotes in medicine are almost all attributed to men. Although women have played many vital roles in the advancement of medicine, they generally did not get their names into the history books. Today, things are changing. In 2003, for the first time in history, women outnumbered men in the first-year classes in U.S. medical schools (1). Of course, it will take time, but eventually women's contributions may come to equal, or even eclipse, those of men.

To streamline the presentation of references, I have used two styles of citations. The first is a shorthand method, included in the text, citing the page number of the source of a fact or short quotation taken from one of the books listed in the Bibliography. On the other hand, when presenting a key concept, disputable assertion, or recent clinical innovation (such as the "wait-and-see prescription" for the treatment of acute otitis media) and when I believe the reader might want to seek more information, a specific citation is included in the reference list at the end of each chapter.

I have spent many hours checking the details presented in this book. I checked the atlas to verify that Miltown (the brand name of the antianxiety agent meprobamate) is indeed named for a small town—Milltown, New Jersey. I have verified that mandrake is mentioned in the Bible (Genesis 30:14–16) as an adjunct to fertility. I have confirmed that an 1884 article on the syndrome of *penis captivus*, attributed to Egerton Yorrick Davis and published in the *Philadelphia Medical News*, was actually a practical joke from the pen of the venerable Sir William Osler.

In spite of all my efforts, I am certain that some readers will dispute various facts in the pages that follow. How could this occur? My careful fact checking led me to two discoveries: First, the experts sometimes disagree. For example, some hold that the disease name "trench mouth" came from *trenchers*, a word used to describe the sometimes wormy wooden plates used for eating in the Middle Ages; others assert that the name arose because of its association with the mud-filled trenches of World War I. Chapter 4 presents my best information as to which is true. Second, there are some inaccuracies in the medical literature, and there is even more misinformation on the Internet, where anyone with access to a Web site can post believable, but not entirely factual, data (without a hint of peer review). And so, valued reader, if you disagree with a fact or two in the book, please let me know and we will do our research together—so that the next edition of the book can be almost perfect. Also, if you know of an interesting item in medical history, a handy clinical adage, or a noteworthy clinical misadventure, please send it along to me.

I have heard the term *organizational culture* described as a shared narrative of a group. Medicine as a profession has its own culture, one that is quite different from that of, for instance, police officers or librarians or farmers. We who practice medicine have our unique shared narrative, comprised of thousands of tales that begin with the ministrations of primitive healers. In a sense, then, this book contains what used to be stories told around the campfire—the exploits of heroes, the misdeeds of rogues, memorable occurrences, humorous events, and a few incredible fables.

In some three-plus millennia of recorded medical history, there have been some profound feats of intellect and some stupefying errors of judgment. And somehow, at the end of these *White Coat Tales*, we come to where we are today in the science and practice of medicine. As to the future, we can be assured only that there will be new stories of how some of today's clinical concepts were either prescient or wrong-headed and that health care in the years ahead will be different than it is today.

Robert B. Taylor, MD
Portland, OR

Reference

1. Barzansky B, Etzel SI. Educational programs in US medical schools, 2003–2004. *JAMA*. 2004;292:1025–1031.

Part One
Heroes, Diseases, and Remedies

1
Heroes in Medical History

You have chosen the most fascinating and dynamic profession there is, a profession with the highest potential for greatness, since the physician's daily work is wrapped up in the subtle web of history. Your labors are linked with those of your colleagues who preceded you in history, and those who are now working all over the world. It is this spiritual unity with our colleagues of all periods and all countries that has made medicine so universal and eternal. For this reason we must study and try to imitate the lives of the "Great Doctors" of history.

Félix Martí-Ibáñez
epilogue to *A Prelude to Medical History* (1)

Medicine has traveled a long and illustrious path over the past millennia, beginning with the first instance when one of our long-forgotten ancestors noticed that a sick or injured person recovered following some earnest appeal to the spirits of nature and culminating in the recent major milestone of the mapping of the human genome. This chapter will take us along that trail as we look in on the lives of the "Great Doctors," the heroes of medical history. As your guide, I will point out only what I believe to be the most significant highlights. The real purpose of this chapter is not to make you a medical historian, but to put medical history in perspective so that the 12 chapters of this book make sense in the context of our heritage.

Beginning the Journey

At this time, let me make a few declarative statements about the chapter, three assertions that I will explain below:

1. This will be a whirlwind trip through the pages of medical history.
2. The chapter will be about persons, dates, and advances in medicine.
3. I make no claim that what is presented here is complete or even that it represents the "most relevant" topics.

An Overview of Key Events

Sadly, most medical school graduates today know precious little about medicine's heroes, heritage, and misadventures. With the astounding proliferation of medical knowledge over recent decades, there has been a growing perception that medical students must learn much more than was taught a generation or two ago—without a corresponding prolongation of medical education. Medical school is still the same four years in duration that it was two generations ago. As a result, some important items have been squeezed from the curriculum; today, young doctors learn little about Ambroise Paré, Edward Jenner, or John Snow. To be fair, they also leave medical school woefully naive about health care policy, medical politics, personal finance, and how to make a living as a doctor. But, the latter deficiencies of current medical education aside, here we will focus on knowing more about this noble profession.

Persons, Medical Advances, and Dates

If I have seen further, it is by standing on the shoulders of giants.

The quotation above is from Isaac Newton (1642–1727), writing to Robert Hooke, scientist and later architect, in 1676. If this chapter is chiefly about any single thing, it is about giants. Although many of the persons described made contributions in diverse areas, most are remembered for one fabled accomplishment, such as William Withering's use of foxglove (digitalis) to treat congestive heart failure. Many were giants because they were acknowledged leaders of their times; in some instances, they also took risks and opposed current thinking, as when Ignaz Semmelweis suggested that doctors' unwashed hands might carry disease.

Because a knowledge of eras and dates is important, I have presented items in chronological order as much as possible, recognizing that not all historians agree on the dates of named eras and that many medical advances evolved during overlapping times. I hope that you, the reader, will strive to learn the chronology, which is how we put things in perspective later in the book.

Completeness and Relevance

Books about medical history tend to be exhaustive and their authors are cautious to include anyone of possible note. There may also be an ever-so-slight bias that depends on the specialty of the author (or lecturer). If the author is a surgeon, you will hear about John Hunter and William S. Halsted; if your lecturer is a public health specialist, expect to learn about James Lind and Louis Pasteur. If you read a number of books or attend several lectures, you will hear of many names and deeds as if all of them were of equal importance. I disagree.

In this chapter, I have been very selective in the persons described. They must have met two criteria: Each must have made a major and enduring contribution to medicine. And the person and his or her achievement must have earned a special niche in the pantheon of medical heroes, so that every 21st century physician *should* know of that individual's life and work.

What follows will seem a little like a sports highlights film—the end-zone reception and the spectacular dunk. However, be assured that if you know the persons, achievements, and dates in this single chapter, you will know far more medical history than most physicians. In addition, if you can spot the epistemological threads among the various advances, you are becoming a bit of a medical historian.

From Superstition to Science

Primitive, Egyptian, Chinese, and Babylonian Medicine

The time of primitive medicine flows gradually into the allegedly more civilized eras described later. The order of presenting Egyptian, Chinese, and Babylonian medicine is somewhat arbitrary, given that these civilizations flourished for long and overlapping times and in different parts of the world.

Primitive Healers and Mind-Body Medicine

Our knowledge of primitive medicine can be deduced only from archeological findings. There were no clearly written records and no known heroes. The beginnings must have been when some tribal member attributed the body's healing powers to some well-intentioned incantation, charm, or spell. Recognized abilities in this regard led to the identification of healers—the first medicine men and women. In time, herbal remedies emerged; probably a few even had beneficial properties. In retrospect, the value of most early medicine was in the belief that something was being done and that a person—the healer—offered hope.

Eventually, there emerged individuals with singular knowledge of natural remedies or expertise in setting broken bones. Then came individuals who developed early surgical techniques and even a form of acupuncture (see below). The march to medical specialization had begun.

Nevertheless, primitive medicine lacked the "evidence-based" *summum bonum* we seek today, and its efficacy relied heavily on the belief in natural remedies which is now being rediscovered under the rubric of integrative health care.

Ancient Egyptian Medicine: A Comprehensive Approach to Medicine
(Beginning ca. 2900 BCE)

Ancient Egypt's "Father of Medicine" is Imhotep, who lived about the 28th century BCE. His name means "He who comes in peace," and he was a philosopher, astronomer, magician, and poet, as well as a physician. Imhotep proposed theories about the roles of vital organs and he diagnosed and treated hundreds of diseases. To him is attributed the saying, "Eat, drink, and be merry for tomorrow we shall die."

Much of what we know about early Egyptian medicine comes from the medical papyri. The Edwin Smith Surgical Papyrus, dating from the 17th century BCE and named for the American Egyptologist who found the document in Luxor, is the oldest known surgical treatise. It lists problems in a systematic way: presentation, physical examination, assessment, and verdict. The verdict in some cases was that "nothing can be done"—a remarkable observation for early healers.

Through the practices of surgery, autopsy, and embalming, the ancient Egyptians came to a reasonable understanding of human anatomy, including the circulatory system. They used trephination for head injuries and filled teeth with a type of mineral cement. They had an extensive pharmacopoeia of remedies for various ailments. In the centuries to follow, Hippocrates and Galen both visited the Temple of Imhotep in Memphis (near today's Cairo) to study the works of Egyptian physicians.

Nothing good lasts forever, and Inglis (p. 21) writes that degeneration "in medical practice is usually closely related to a decline of a national culture; and so it was in Egypt." In the fifth century BCE, the historian Herodotus visited Egypt, describing its medical system as bloated with specialists vying for access to various body parts. As a medical educator, I wonder whether there is a parallel to the large number of students entering medical school today aspiring to become subspecialists.

Ancient Chinese Medicine: Herbal Treatment and Acupuncture
(Beginning ca. 2700 BCE)

It seems that every system of medicine requires a "Father" or (in the phrase of Martí-Ibáñez) a Great Doctor. According to Garrison (p. 73), the founder of ancient Chinese medicine is the emperor Shen Nung (ca. 2737 BCE), who wrote the herbal *Pen Tsao*. This book described a number of botanical remedies, one of which is a compound from which ephedrine is derived.

We can trace acupuncture in Chinese medicine back to the time of the Stone Age, and Inglis (p. 13) suggests that "above the folklore level there is no other direct link with early medicine." Acupuncture—then and now—is based on maintaining balance among the forces of *yang* and *yin*—representing plus and minus, light and dark. This quest to achieve balance is a recurring theme in ancient Chinese medicine.

Ancient Babylonian Medicine: The Code of Hammurabi (Beginning ca. 2250 BCE)

By the third century BCE, medicine in Babylon had, according to the Hammurabi Code, become regulated by government. Fees for various types of care were set by law, taking into consideration the patient's ability to pay. A gentleman paid 10 shekels in silver to have a wound treated, whereas a poor man, with the same wound, paid half that amount.

Government control had some perils for physicians. If a physician's error caused the patient to lose an eye, the doctor might also lose an eye.

Greco-Roman Medicine (ca. Fifth Century BCE–Fifth Century CE)

It seems appropriate to begin the tale of Greco-Roman medicine with Aesculapius, even though he probably lived only in legend. He was the son of Apollo and Coronis and was taught medicine and, notably, surgery by the centaur Chiron. The staff of Aesculapius was entwined with a single snake, and I will return to this in chapter 11. He had six daughters, of whom three were named Panacea (literally, "all-healing"), Hygieia ("cleanliness"), and Meditrine ("medicine"). The name of one of his sons, Telesforos, suggests "recuperation." Legend holds that Aesculapius was born a mortal but later became a god. In the end, he angered Zeus, who killed him with a thunderbolt.

Aesculapius shows up often in history and literature. Centers of healing, called *aesculapia*, were established at a number of sites in Greece, notably Epidaurus and the Island of Kos. Aesculapius is mentioned in the first line of the classic Hippocratic Oath, and Socrates' final words were a request to Crito to sacrifice a cock to Aesculapius; Socrates, believing that his spirit would shortly depart for the joys of the blessed, wished to thank the god of medicine for the cup of hemlock he had just drunk.

Ancient Grecian Medicine: Hippocrates and Scientific Observation (Beginning ca. 460–377 BCE)

Although we are not quite sure of Aesculapius' mortality, Hippocrates certainly lived (1). Born on the Island of Kos in 460 BCE, Hippocrates believed that hygienic methods and proper diet could enhance a patient's vitality. He and his disciples used critical observation and deductive reasoning to break the bond between mysticism and medicine. Hippocrates reportedly received the sick under the shade of a plane tree (a type of sycamore), the arboreal descendent of which still exists today in a quiet village square on the Island of Kos. On a hillside outside of the village is the Temple of Aesculapius, where Hippocrates and his colleagues healed, taught, and recorded their observations—making the site arguably the world's first academic medical center. Today, some families on the Island of Kos claim that they are descendants of Hippocrates.

Some 70 works comprise the Hippocratic Corpus, writings attributed to Hippocrates. What is not certain is that Hippocrates actually wrote them (2). I will return to the authorship issue in chapter 10. Some of the most pertinent Hippocratic observations were stated as aphorisms, which are discussed in chapter 7 (3).

In 377 BCE, in the words of Marcus Aurelius, "Hippocrates, after curing many diseases, himself fell sick and died" (4).

Ancient Roman Medicine: Public Health Measures (ca. First Century BCE–500 CE)

Although there was some penetration of Greek medicine into Roman life, Romans generally seemed to ignore much of the medical knowledge of their day. They believed themselves to be indestructible and considered the Greeks and their medicine to be effete. "No-nonsense Roman tradition held that one was better off without doctors," writes Porter (p. 69). Garrison (p. 117) is even more critical: "Of the condition of medicine under the Romans considerable is known but little need be said."

On the other hand, we must laud the ancient Romans for one singular advance—their keen attention to public health measures. They valued personal cleanliness and physical exercise. They worked to ensure pure water by building a system of aqueducts, some spanning many miles. They constructed elaborate public baths, and they built drains and sewers to remove waste. They espoused cremation of the dead. But, again according to Garrison, they did so as part of the cult of Vesta and Juturna, producing "hygienic results without medical intention" (p. 120).

The luminary—more or less—of ancient Roman medicine was Claudius Galen.

Galenic System of Medicine: Claudius Galen (129–200 CE)

Porter (p. 71) calls Galen "the medical colossus of the Roman era." What did Galen do to merit such an accolade? Galen was a student of medicine and did his best to pass on his findings. Early in his career, he was a physician to gladiators, giving him the opportunity to examine the workings of the human body at a time when human dissection was forbidden. He dissected a wide variety of animals—pigs, dogs, and monkeys. He described cardiac arrhythmias and the use of the pulse in diagnosis. He recorded his observations, and he systematized virtually all the medical knowledge of his time in hundreds of written works, some 200 of which survive today. There was only one problem.

Much of what Galen wrote was wrong. For example, he concluded that the human heart has only two chambers. He believed that humans, like dogs, have five-lobed livers. He believed that the brain secreted a "vital spirit" that was carried via hollow nerves to the muscles, permitting movement. Inglis (p. 39) cites a critic of Galen who describes his works as "a weird hodgepodge of nonsense, Aristotelian philosophy, Hippocratic dogma, and shrewd clinical and experimental observations."

Now, none of this would have been so bad, and Galenic medicine would have been just another step in the march of medicine, had it not been for one noteworthy historical event. Sometime around the fall of the Eastern Roman Empire in 476 CE, the world descended into the Dark Ages. As a result of this turning point in history, Galen's collection of insightful truths and deductive errors became the recognized medical authority for a millennium. In the words of Cartwright (p. 27), "If Christ was the founder of the Christian school of medicine, Galen was its acknowledged authority and unchallenged teacher." Small wonder he is considered immensely influential and, at the same time, a misleading force in the history of medicine.

The Middle Ages (Fifth to 14th Century)

The Middle Ages, aka medieval times, describes a period in Western European history which roughly begins with the fall of the Roman Empire in the fifth century and ends with the beginning of the Renaissance in the 14th century and the subsequent discovery of the New World. The Dark Ages refers to the Early Middle Ages, beginning about the middle of the fifth century and lasting for 300 years, the period of greatest medieval intellectual stagnation—at least in most of Europe. With the fall of Roman civilization, the Church became the custodian of Western scholarship. The warfare and general turmoil in continental Europe prompted historian Thomas Cahill to write a book entitled *How the Irish Saved Civilization*, describing how Christian monks in Ireland transcribed classical texts that were in danger following the fall of Rome (5). The title may be a bit hyperbolic, but it conveys the tenor of early medieval times.

Two institutions shaped the Middle Ages. The first was feudalism, with an agricultural economy and tenant farmers dominated by lords of the manor. The second was Christianity, the tenets of which permeated all aspects of medieval life.

The Middle Ages were, to be charitable, a quiet time in the history of medicine. In the words of Inglis (p. 49), "After Galen's death progress ceased, and medicine regressed into sorcery. Only at the Renaissance was progress resumed; only at the Renaissance, therefore, does medical history become significant once more." This is not to say that there were no medieval healers. There were many, using herbs and leeches, religion and mysticism. Yet despite challenges such as the Black Death (bubonic plague), which wiped out a quarter of Europe's population in the late 1340s, there were no noteworthy advances and no giants—at least in Europe.

What were dark times in Europe became a golden age to the east.

Critical Observation: Rhazes (850–923)

Born in Persia, Abū Bakr Muhammad ibn Zakarīya al-Rāzi was known to the Europeans as Rhazes. He was one of the major philosophers of Islam and wrote some 200 books, including 25 volumes describing his medical observations. Versed in the Hippocratic approach, Rhazes challenged Galenic dogma. His writings disagree with Galen's description of the course of a fever. He differentiated among the spotted fevers, such as measles and smallpox. Rhazes advocated a sound mind in a sound body and wrote of the importance of the patient-physician relationship.

Systemization of Medicine: Avicenna (980–1037)

The author of some 450 books on a variety of topics, Persian physician and philosopher Avicenna earned a place among the Great Doctors by writing a million-word, five-volume *Canon of Medicine*. This book, which sought to reconcile Galen's theories with Aristotelian teachings, has been called "perhaps the most studied medical work ever written" (Martí-Ibáñez, p. 112).

Scholarly Approach to Disease: Moses Maimonides (1135–1204)

Moses Maimonides was one of the most prolific authors of the Middle Ages and the shining star of Jewish physicians of the time. Sir William Osler once described him as "the Prince of Physicians" (6). Maimonides wrote 10 medical books. His works include *Extracts from Galen* and *Commentary on the Aphorisms of Hippocrates*. In the latter book, according to Rosner, Hippocrates is reported to have stated, "A boy is born from the right ovary, a girl from the left." Maimonides comments that "a man would have to be either prophet or genius to know this" (6).

Maimonides' other works include *Asthma*, *Explanation of Fits*, *Poisons and Their Antidotes*, *Hemorrhoids*, *Cohabitation*, *Regimen of Health*, and *Drug Names*. His *Medical Aphorisms of Moses Maimonides* contains some 1,500 succinct observations, some of which are presented in chapter 7 of this book.

The Renaissance and Reformation (15th and 16th Centuries)

In high school, we learned that the Renaissance began in Italy in the 15th century and subsequently spread across Europe. Inglis (p. 72) suggests a specific birth date, 1443, the year of the discovery of the manuscript *De Re Medicina*, part of Celsus' encyclopedia. The manuscript, found in a Milan church, had been lost since Roman times. The Renaissance—the time of Leonardo da Vinci, Niccolò Machiavelli, and Raphael—was followed by the

Reformation, a 16th century religious rebellion against Roman Catholic dogmatism. Three medical giants dominated these eras: Paracelsus, Paré, and Vesalius.

Iatrochemistry: Paracelsus (1493–1542)

Swiss physician Theophrastus Bombast von Hohenheim took the name Paracelsus; Dirckx (p. 46) believes the name was chosen to assert that his work went beyond that of Celsus. Osler, who had a penchant for epithets, termed him "the [Martin] Luther of medicine; the very incarnation of revolt" (Inglis, p. 72). In 1527, just to emphasize his spirit of revolt, Paracelsus publicly torched the medieval works of Middle Eastern physician Avicenna and of the controversial Galen.

So what did Paracelsus contribute? He postulated a "life force" and asserted that nature was the ruling power whom the physician was obliged to understand and obey (Porter, p. 202). Curiously, given this premise, he postulated a system based on chemical principles, with the chief substances identified as sulfur, mercury, and salt. He also went on to take a new look at old diseases, such as gout.

Inglis (p. 73) holds that, of all the diverse disciplines that owe a debt to Paracelsus, the greatest benefit has been to psychiatry. He held that "the character of the physician acts more powerfully upon the patient than all the drugs administered," presaging the statement by Michael Balint some four centuries later that in many cases "the doctor is the drug" (7).

Thus, it is ironic that some remember Paracelsus best for his attention to chemistry. Perhaps, this is because most of Paracelsus' writings were published after his death in 1542 and many of those who followed focused on his attention to chemistry, giving rise to what Porter (p. 209) calls Paracelsan iatrochemistry.

Wound Care: Ambroise Paré (ca. 1517–1564)

In contrast to Paracelsus, Ambroise Paré earned his place in the list of heroes by a single act. He was trained as a barber-surgeon and treated many victims of gunshot wounds. Like the surgeons of his day, he believed that gunpowder was poisonous and that gunshot wounds should be cauterized by a mixture of boiling oil and salve. Then one day, following an especially bloody battle during the siege of Turin in 1537, the supply of oil ran out. With no boiling oil, the remaining injuries were treated with a cold mixture of egg yolk, turpentine, and oil of roses. Paré noted that the wounds treated without boiling oil recovered more rapidly than those doused with boiling oil, changing the course of wound care forever.

As might be expected, not all welcomed Paré's findings enthusiastically. The medical faculty in Paris disparaged his writings as not only contradictory to current belief but written in a vernacular that was not at all scholarly.

Fortunately, reason prevailed, and Paré's work in wound care and other areas led to the greatest advances in surgery until the introduction of asepsis and anesthesia in the 19th century.

Anatomic Dissection: Vesalius (1514–1564)

If psychiatry was advanced by Paracelsus, anatomy must acknowledge an even greater debt to Vesalius, who, Garrison (p. 218) asserts, "alone made anatomy what it is today—a living, working science." Vesalius was the pro-sector at the medical school in Padua, where he revolutionized the physical layout of the medical classroom, bringing students close to the dissection in an amphitheater that still exists today. He and his students studied the human body in situ, revolutionary in its time.

In 1543, Vesalius published *De Humani Corporis Fabrica*, an anatomically precise and liberally illustrated textbook of anatomy. He, like others, refuted Galenic dogma, showing that the heart has four chambers, not two.

I wish I could say that the pioneering book was well received, but such was not the case. He and his work were highly criticized, even by Vesalius' mentor, Sylvius. Colleagues sought to discredit him. In a rage, Vesalius burned his manuscripts and departed Padua for Madrid, where he became a courtier and abandoned the study of anatomy forever.

The Seventeenth Century

The 1600s were a vibrant century. It was the time of Baroque art, the James-town settlement in the New World, the Dutch tulip mania, and the end of the Thirty Years' War. These hundred years were the time of Francis Bacon and William Shakespeare in England, Jean Racine and Moliére in France, Rembrandt van Rijn in Holland, and Miguel de Cervantes in Spain. During this century, ice cream was invented, the speed of light was first measured, and bullbaiting was a popular recreational activity in England.

During this time, there were three very significant advances in medicine.

Circulation of the Blood: William Harvey (1578–1657)

William Harvey plunged the final dagger into Galenic theory. Although born in England, Harvey studied at Padua, undoubtedly in the dissection amphitheater of Vesalius. He earned another medical degree at Cambridge University before beginning medical practice.

Harvey deduced that the heart pumped the blood, which circulated through the lungs and the body before returning to the heart for recircula-tion. This was quite different form Galenic theory, which held that there were two types of blood, arterial and venous, which never mingled, and that food was converted into blood by the liver and subsequently used as fuel by the body.

In 1628, Harvey published *Exercitatio Anatomica du Motu Cordis et Sanguinis in Animalibus* (An Anatomical Essay Concerning the Movement of the Heart and Blood in Animals). As might be predicted, Galenic stalwarts attacked Harvey. As Porter writes (p. 216), "It would mean, for instance, that the liver was no longer the blood-making organ, and once the liver's function was questioned, what else would not be questioned?" But Harvey survived the assault and prevailed to become the physician to the court of Charles I of England and to be recognized as a medical giant during his lifetime.

Classic Descriptions of Disease: Thomas Sydenham (1624–1689)

Sometimes called "the English Hippocrates," Thomas Sydenham resurrected the Hippocratic methods of observation and deduction (Garrison, p. 269). He also suffered from gout, and his writing on gout has been considered his finest work, despite his rejection of colchicine as a safe remedy. Today, he is best known for his insightful descriptions of diseases, some of which were dysentery, hysteria, pneumonitis, measles, scarlatina, malarial fevers, and chorea (sometimes called Sydenham chorea).

In remembering his contributions to diagnosis, we should not forget his therapeutic insights: the value of Peruvian bark (a source of quinine) for malaria, the advocacy of fresh air in sickrooms, and the benefits of Sydenham's Laudanum—a mixture of sherry wine, herbs, and opium.

Sydenham has been described as bringing doctors out of the laboratory and into the sickroom and subsequently sending clinical researchers back to the laboratories to explain the illnesses they encountered (Inglis, p. 101).

The Discovery of Microorganisms: Anton van Leeuwenhoek (1632–1723)

At the outset, let us be clear that van Leeuwenhoek did not invent the microscope. Zacharias Janssen in Holland, probably with the help of his father, is given credit for building the first compound microscope (around 1595). Robert Hooke used the microscope to study, among other things, lice. Hooke first used the word "cell" in a scientific sense, referring to the "pores" in wood (Porter, p. 223). Later, in Pisa, Marcello Malpighi studied the tongue, the blood, and internal viscera, leaving his name strewn eponymously throughout human anatomy.

But we remember van Leeuwenhoek, and we do so because he was the first to describe microorganisms, which he called *animicules*. He observed a wide variety of tiny living things, including bacteria, protozoa, and human spermatozoa, and in 1673 he published his findings in the Royal Society's *Philosophical Transactions*.

During his lifetime, van Leeuwenhoek built some 400 microscopes, of which 9 exist today. He presented his work to the English Royal Society and, despite some ups and downs, lived to see his work validated by scholars of his time.

His lasting contribution was, of course, that there are tiny organisms, visible only microscopically, that live, multiply, and perhaps have other roles in nature. Later, we would learn that they could be the cause of great mischief.

The Eighteenth Century

During the 1700s, the world experienced the end of the reign of Louis XIV in France and George III assumed the throne of England (in 1760), with implications for the revolt of American colonists which would follow later. The French Revolution of 1789–1799 brought a tumultuous decade to a close. Familiar names from the century included Marie Antoinette and Napoleon Bonaparte, Wolfgang Amadeus Mozart and Johann Sebastian Bach, Queen Anne of England and British navigator James Cook, Scottish poet Robert Burns, and a long list of Founding Fathers of the United States of America.

In medicine, we were expanding our knowledge of some specific diseases and what to do about them.

Prevention of Scurvy: James Lind (1716–1794)

James Lind's contribution was concentrated in one specific area, but it was very important. His work set the stage for prevention of a devastating, but easily avoidable, disease while following a model of controlled clinical experimentation and providing British sailors with an enduring nickname.

In Lind's day, scurvy was common among seamen on long voyages; the longer the voyage, the greater the risk. Lind theorized that citrus fruits might prevent scurvy, although his reasoning was physiologically incorrect; he thought the fundamental problem was faulty digestion. In 1754, aboard the HMS *Salisbury*, Lind conducted an experiment on 12 men with scurvy; two received oranges and lemons, while others were treated with various items, such as vinegar, seawater, oil of vitriol, and a concoction of garlic, radish, myrrh, and balsam of Peru. The two sailors who received the citrus fruit recovered promptly and were then recruited to nurse the other patients (Porter, p. 295).

In 1753, Lind published his findings in *A Treatise of the Scurvy*, but it took some time for his findings to be translated into practice. Eventually, citrus fruits became part of the diet at sea. One of the fruits used was lime, giving rise to the term "limey" for the British seaman.

Surgery as an Experimental Science: John Hunter (1728–1793)

If Lind's achievement was a rifle shot, John Hunter's was a cannon blast. Garrison (p. 347) ranks Hunter as one of the three greatest surgeons of all time, along with Paré and Joseph Lister. Garrison writes, "It is no exaggeration to repeat that Hunter found surgery a mechanical art and left it an experimental science." Moore calls him the "Father of Modern Surgery" (8). Remember that, in Hunter's day, the barber-surgeon had not yet waned and those who cut were called "Mr.," and not "Dr."

A bit of Hunter's aura must come from the colorful legends that whirl about his memory. He dissected countless cadavers, some provided by professional grave robbers. After rupturing his Achilles tendon, Hunter severed the tendons of several dogs, sacrificing them at intervals to observe how the tendon healed. He lacked tact and often lost control of his temper. Moore suggests that he may have been the inspiration for early depictions of the mad scientist (8). More colorful Hunterian stories are found later in the book; here, we will note his accomplishments.

What exactly did Hunter do to deserve high praise?

He was a researcher and innovator. He experimented with bone growth and remodeling, collateral circulation, and tooth transplantation. He devised a tube that could be passed into the stomach to allow artificial feeding and devised an early version of mechanical ventilation. He introduced novel techniques of vascular surgery, said by Garrison (p. 347) to have saved "thousands of limbs and lives."

In the valedictory address at Harvard Commencement on March 10, 1858, Oliver Wendell Holmes stated, "For faithful lifelong study of science you will find no better example than John Hunter, never satisfied until he had the pericardium of Nature open and her heart throbbing naked in his hand" (Strauss, p. 422).

Digitalis Therapy of Dropsy: William Withering (1741–1799)

William Withering was not merely a country doctor. He was a colleague of James Watt (inventor of the steam engine) and Joseph Priestley (the chemist who discovered oxygen). He owned the first water closet in the city of Birmingham, England.

Withering had the humility to listen to his patients. A botanist as well as physician, Withering was intrigued when he heard of a local woman—some say a gypsy—who brewed a tea based on a secret family recipe which could be used to treat dropsy (congestive heart failure). Withering hunted her down and convinced her to share the recipe. He concluded that the active ingredient was foxglove—the leaves of which are known today as a source of digitalis. After various experiments, he gave foxglove tea to a 50-year-old man with severe dropsy in 1775. The patient improved markedly, and Withering reported his findings in 1785 as *An Account of the Foxglove and Some of its Medical Uses*.

After a long illness, Withering died in 1799. On the monument marking his grave in Birmingham is the image of a foxglove plant.

Smallpox Vaccination: Edward Jenner (1749–1823)

Today, with smallpox eradicated from the world (except in selected clinical laboratories), it is hard to imagine the impact of the disease before the age of vaccination. I will tell the tale of smallpox as a disease in chapter 2; here, I will give a single example. In 1721–1722, during an epidemic in Boston, of a total population of 11,000 persons, 6,000 contracted the disease and 800 died. The survivors generally had lifelong scars as souvenirs of their infection (9).

Edward Jenner was not the first to devise a means of preventing smallpox. For 1,000 years, the Chinese had practiced a method of inoculation; smallpox scales were dried and ground to a powder, which was then inhaled. In a method devised later, liquid from a pustule was introduced into a scratch. As early as 1717, Lady Mary Wortley Montagu, wife of the British Ambassador at Constantinople, described the method in a letter home to a friend.

But using live smallpox—called variolation—was clearly dangerous, and the world awaited a safe, and reliable, method of preventing "the speckled monster."

Probably the belief that persons who have suffered cowpox are protected from smallpox had long been a folk legend—awaiting an astute and courageous physician to introduce a useful application into medical practice. Jenner, a physician in the village of Berkeley, Gloucestershire, England, treated a local milkmaid who boasted that she would be safe from smallpox because she had had cowpox. In 1796, Jenner took secretions from an active cowpox lesion and inoculated the arms of a young boy named James Phipps. The boy developed a mild fever, but no severe disease.

As was typical of the medical establishment, the Royal Society scorned Jenner's account of his "vaccination" (taking the word root from *vaca*, meaning cow). But Jenner persisted, and in 1798 he published a pamphlet, *An Inquiry into the Causes and Effects of Variolae Vaccinae, a disease discovered in some of the Western Counties of England, particularly Gloucestershire, and known by the name Cowpox.* With this effort, his work was recognized to the extent that 1803 saw the establishment of the Royal Jennerian Society to promote vaccination. A new age of infectious disease prevention had begun.

In an 1806 letter to Jenner, U.S. President Thomas Jefferson wrote, "Medicine has never before produced any single improvement of such utility. . . . You have erased from the calendar of human afflictions one of its greatest. Yours is the comfortable reflection that mankind can never forget that you have lived. Future nations will know by history only that the loathsome smallpox has existed and by you been extirpated."

Almost as though he were oblivious to his achievements, Jenner continued to live and practice in the village of Berkeley, where he eventually died (Martí-Ibáñez, p. 162).

The Nineteenth Century

When I think of the 19th century, I think of the War of 1812, the American Civil War, and General Custer's foolhardy escapade at the Little Big Horn. I also think of the remarkable persons who lived and worked in the 1800s: Paul Cézanne, Johannes Brahms, Gilbert and Sullivan, Emily Dickinson, Charles Darwin, Jane Austen, Robert E. Lee, and Abraham Lincoln. Public buses, department stores, the game of basketball, and the internal combustion engine would all begin during this century.

In medicine, I think of the following Great Doctors and their contributions: Morton, Semmelweis, Snow, Pasteur, Lister, Roentgen, the Curies, and Osler.

Ether Anesthesia: William T.G. Morton (1819–1868)

Paré brought wound care out of the dark ages. Hunter developed new surgical techniques. The world awaited a method by which surgery—such as the thousands of amputations performed by battlefield surgeons—could be accomplished without excruciating pain. William T.G. Morton, building on some previous work, developed this method.

Morton was a dentist who became interested in the effects of ether, in part after learning about "ether frolics," an activity popular among some pleasure-seekers of the time. In 1846, following experiments on his dog, a dental patient, and then on himself, Morton somehow persuaded his colleagues at Boston's Massachusetts General Hospital to allow him to demonstrate general anesthesia using ether. The patient was a 20-year-old man with a neck tumor. Morton administered the ether, the patient promptly became anesthetized, and Morton exclaimed to the surgeon, "Your patient is ready, sir." Today, the operating room where this took place is called the "Ether Dome."

I wish the story ended there, with Morton receiving well-deserved accolades and honor. Alas, he chose to seek wealth, using his discovery. He added coloring to the gas and announced the discovery of a new agent. He later sought a patent on ether. He lost the respect of his colleagues, and his entrepreneurial and legal adventures were costly. He died in poverty at age 49, leaving his wife and five children penniless. Porter (p. 367) reports that Morton and his fate are an example of "the commercial opportunism bedeviling medicine at that time, especially in America."

Hand Washing: Ignaz Philipp Semmelweis (1818–1865)

Today, medical students dutifully wash their hands before any physical examination, and surgeons "scrub up" before entering the operating room. In the early 19th century, hand washing was not part of the clinician's routine. Viennese obstetrician Ignaz Semmelweis observed that medical students often came from performing autopsies to attend women in childbirth without attention to personal cleanliness. Their patients had a high incidence of "childbed fever," much higher than another ward staffed by midwifery students. Semmelweis had them exchange locations; the medical students' patients continued to have a higher incidence of infection. Could the cause be contaminated material from the autopsy room? This question was prescient, because although van Leeuwenhoek had observed microorganisms in the 17th century, the germ theory of disease was yet to come.

In May 1847, Semmelweis ordered both medical and midwifery students to wash their hands with chlorinated water prior to deliveries. The rates of infection in both wards fell. We would all rejoice if the merits of his discovery were instantly recognized and surgeons had promptly adopted the hand-washing technique. However, there was the by-now predictable opposition to change, and in the words of Nuland, "Semmelweis' story has come down to us as Exhibit A in the case for obstinacy and blindness of physicians" (10). He lost his position in Vienna and moved to Budapest, where he would loudly criticize any physician who failed to scrub up. In the end, he developed a psychiatric illness, was admitted to a mental hospital, and ironically died of sepsis following a finger infection, perhaps caused by the same organism that caused childbed fever (Sebastian, pp. 659–660).

Public Health Activism: John Snow (1813–1858)

A single day—one act—secured for John Snow his place in history. Although a surgeon and "London's leading anesthesiologist" (Porter, p. 412), Snow became interested in cholera as an epidemic swept through London.

During an especially severe outbreak in the Soho district in 1854, Snow observed that in a single week, many cholera deaths occurred in townspeople drinking water from the Broad Street pump. Persons drinking water from other sources had a much lower incidence of cholera. Snow convinced the Board of Guardians of St. James Parish, home of the Broad Street pump, that the pump must be dismantled. Snow wrote, "In consequence of what I said, the handle of the pump was removed the following day."

After the removal of the pump handle, there was a steep decline in cholera cases in the neighborhood. Snow had demonstrated that the pump water was the source of cholera. Then, in 1855, he spoke to the House of Commons Select Committee, and he played a role in decisions that led to improvements in the water supply and sewage systems in London.

Snow thus accomplished two things: He demonstrated that cholera was, in this instance, waterborne and not caused by "miasmata." Also, he demonstrated the gains that can be achieved by public health activism—foreshadowing methods to be used later in the battles against tobacco, obesity, and drunk driving. In March 2003, a survey by *Hospital Doctor* magazine voted John Snow the "greatest doctor of all time." The magazine's readers ranked Hippocrates as number two.

Germ Theory of Disease: Louis Pasteur (1822–1895)

By the second half of the 19th century, physician-scientists knew about microorganisms, about how small doses of an infection can prevent the full-blown disease, and how vehicles (such as water) can carry infection (such as cholera). Louis Pasteur connected the dots, postulating the "germ theory of disease" and developing vaccines against anthrax, cholera, and rabies.

He also discovered that partial heat sterilization (pasteurization) could prevent the spoilage of wine and beer. A nationalistic citizen of France, Pasteur went on to patent a beer-making process with the intent of outshining the "scoundrelly Germans." Pasteur's beverage was to be marketed as the "Beer of Revenge."

Pasteur is quoted as saying, "When meditating over a disease, I never think of finding a remedy for it, but, instead, a means to prevent it." Pasteur's early work involved immunization in chickens, sheep, and cattle. In 1885, however, his rabies vaccine received a human test when a rabid dog bit an Alsatian boy, Joseph Meister. The bite was treated successfully with the vaccine, and three years late the Pasteur Institute was opened in Paris.

Perhaps the most famous quote attributed to Pasteur is this: "Did you ever observe to whom the accidents happen? Chance only favors the prepared mind" (Strauss, p. 108).

Surgical Antisepsis: Joseph Lister (1827–1912)

Over the years, surgical techniques continued to be refined, pain-free operations under general anesthesia became possible, physicians came to value the simple act of hand washing, and the world learned about germs. Joseph Lister, familiar with Pasteur's work, wondered whether airborne germs might be a cause of surgical infections. His solution in 1866 was to spray the surgical field with a solution of carbolic acid, a compound chosen because it reduced the odor of lands irrigated with sewage and the "entozoa" that infested cattle fed in pastures near the town of Carlisle, England.

His theory was laudable, but carbolic acid (phenol) soon was found to be excessively caustic. Boric acid was a better choice, but the principle of using chemicals to destroy germs had been established.

The discipline awaited the next innovation—the introduction of surgical gloves by William S. Halsted in 1890.

X-rays Discovered: Wilhelm Conrad Roentgen (1845–1922)

Wilhelm Roentgen made a focused contribution to medicine, one that eventually earned him the 1901 Nobel Prize in Physics. In November 1895, Roentgen, a physics professor, was testing cathode rays in a darkened room. Having screened the tube with black cardboard to block the light it emitted, he was surprised to see a fluorescent screen nearby glow with a green color. Some sort of previously unrecognized emission (which he came to call the x-ray) had passed through the cardboard. Roentgen grasped the significance of his discovery. To test it further, he beamed the rays through his wife's hand and noted the outline of the bones and flesh on the screen beyond.

In contrast to many of the witnesses of other discoveries in history, Roentgen's colleagues lauded his finding and quickly devised clinical applications. On January 7, 1896, the first clinical radiograph was taken, setting the stage for a whole new medical specialty.

Discovery of Radium: Marie Curie (1867–1934) and Pierre Curie (1859–1906)

In 1898, while working in Paris, Marie and Pierre Curie discovered radium. They worked first with thorium and uranium by-products, and they coined the term "radioactive." On their road to discovery, Marie handled huge quantities of minerals while Pierre used his own skin to test the effects of radium.

In 1903, the Curies received the Nobel Prize in Physics. Three years later, Pierre was killed in an automobile accident, whereas Marie lived until 1934, when at age 67, she died of leukemia, almost certainly caused by "her" radium. She lived long enough, however, to witness the medical application of radioactive agents to treat cancer.

Patient-Centered Medicine: William Osler (1849–1919)

In a few short paragraphs, what shall I select to present about William Osler, a towering figure whose career linked the 19th and 20th centuries? I recall reading somewhere (I cannot find the source) that there have been more words written *about* Sir William than he himself wrote during his lifetime, no small feat considering that he was a prolific author who published hundreds of articles. His most tangible achievement was the textbook *The Principles and Practice of Medicine*, which was published in 1892 and endured through 16 editions until 1947. He was an inveterate bibliophile who once wrote, "It is astonishing with how little reading a doctor can practice medicine, but it is not astonishing how badly he may do it."

Certainly, he was the physician's role model of a role model. Beighton (p. 131) writes, "He had a profound influence on many young physicians who later achieved eminence and this aspect of his work is widely regarded as his greatest achievement."

I believe that Osler's enduring contribution was his advocacy for—and role modeling of—patient-centered medicine. Legend holds that once, while attired in his academic regalia, Osler peeled and cut a peach, which he fed to a child with whooping cough. Osler's *Aphorisms* clearly reflects his humanism and his respect for patients as people; I refer to this work and his aphorisms in chapter 7. His humanity shines clearly in his famous addresses, collected in the book *Aequanimitas with Other Addresses to Medical Students, Nurses and Practitioners of Medicine*, which was given to medical students by Eli Lilly & Company until about 1953 (11). In fact, in my personal, well-worn copy is a letter signed "Eli Lilly, President." In the address "Unity, Peace and Concord," Osler ends with "a single word that is my parting commandment." The word is *charity*.

The Twentieth Century

All adults reading this book were alive during the 20th century. Because of advances in communication, transportation, and ways to kill one another, the 1900s witnessed more changes in the world than any previous century. Epic events were World Wars I and II and a host of regional conflicts. Innovations included the assembly line, air travel, and nuclear fission. We recall many influential figures of the times, including Winston Churchill, Juan and Eva Perón, Adolf Hitler, Joseph Stalin, Charles de Gaulle, Mao Zedong, Martin Luther King, and a host of American presidents. In sports and the arts, just a few of the standouts were Pablo Picasso, Marilyn Monroe, Orson Welles, Ayn Rand, Muhammad Ali, Joe Namath, and Madonna.

During all of this, medicine made huge strides in assorted areas such as psychotherapy, medical education reform, prevention of deficiency diseases, hormone replacement, antibiotic therapy, disease prevention, and the recognition of a new but very formidable disease entity—human immunodeficiency virus (HIV) and the acquired immunodeficiency syndrome (AIDS).

Legitimization of Psychiatry: Sigmund Freud (1856–1939)

Paracelsus may have set the stage for the emergence of psychiatry, but the physician who elucidated many of the defining theories of the discipline was Sigmund Freud.

The work of Freud, somehow appropriately, spans the end of the 19th and the beginning of the 20th century. Freud was a very complicated man. He had phobias, including a profound fear of death. He did some early studies of hypnotism. His recollections of sexual feelings for his mother during childhood formed the groundwork for what he would later name "the Oedipus complex." He smoked cigars and continued to do so even after contracting cancer of the oral cavity. He misused cocaine, which I discuss in more detail in chapter 11. In the end, Freud's death from a large dose of morphine was an early instance of physician-assisted suicide.

Perhaps his complicated personality engendered creativity. Freud was a neurologist by training and did important work on cerebral palsy before turning to the intricacies of the human psyche. Today considered the "Father of Psychoanalysis," Freud developed theories of the unconscious mind and of dreams as a source of insight into the unconscious mind. From his work came concepts such as repression, defense mechanisms, transference, libido, and sublimation. Freud set the stage for the development of psychiatry as the specialty we know today.

The First "Magic Bullet": Paul Ehrlich (1854–1915)

Paul Ehrlich, at the Royal Prussian Institute for Experimental Therapy at Frankfort-am-Main, Germany, may have had an especially keen interest in the chemotherapy of disease, since he had found tubercle bacilli in his own sputum. Ehrlich's vision was an arsenal of specific drugs for specific diseases, a dream earlier held by Paracelsus and Sydenham. By Ehrlich's time, however, we knew of germs and toxins, and the quest for the "magic bullet" seemed within reach. Following work with a number of disease treatments—methylene blue for malaria and arsenical compounds for trypanosomiasis—he turned his attention to syphilis.

In the next chapter, I will tell the saga of syphilis through the ages. For now, be aware that by the first decade of the 20th century, the cause of the disease (*Treponema pallidum*) had been identified and a diagnostic blood test (the Wasserman test) was available. Ehrlich set out to find the cure.

Ehrlich continued his work with arsenicals, testing more than 600 compounds. In 1907, arsenical compound number 606 seemed to be especially effective, and work focused on this substance. The compound came to be known as Salvarsan, and within 3 years, more than 10,000 syphilitic patients had been treated. In time, the drug proved to be unacceptably toxic and not as effective as originally believed. In 1914, a new formulation, Neo-Salvarsan, was introduced.

Despite the fact that, in the long run, neither formulation was as useful or as safe as had been hoped, Ehrlich's remedies were the best hope for syphilis victims at the time, prompting physician-journalist Victor Robinson to refer to Ehrlich as "a savior of the race" (Inglis, p. 160).

U.S. Medical Education Reform: Abraham Flexner (1866–1959)

In 1910, the Carnegie Foundation for the Advancement of Teaching published *Medical Education in the United States and Canada*. The "Flexner Report" led to sweeping changes in medical education across North America. The context for Flexner's work was the 19th century effort to exert government control over who could practice medicine. Shryock (p. 140) writes, "In 1821, for example, a Georgia law restricted practice to men holding a degree. Legislation of this sort, when enforced at all, was less likely to raise standards than it was to encourage the founding of easy schools." In other states such as New York and Massachusetts, medical schools were granted licensing powers, and many of these schools did not maintain high standards.

In the report, Flexner deplored the state of U.S. medical education in many schools of his day, citing the anatomy laboratory at one institution as an "outhouse, whence the noisome odor of decaying cadavers permeates the premises" and another school that was "dirty and disorderly beyond repair." He advocated a medical school with professors engaged in research and teaching, and he clearly favored education that began with the first two years dedicated to laboratory studies. The clear message was that we needed fewer, but better, medical schools. Flexner advocated that the number of U.S. medical schools be reduced from 155 to 31 and that the annual number of graduating physicians drop to 2,000 from the then-current total of 4,442 (12).

The outcome was the closure of a number of U.S. medical schools. By 1920, 76 U.S. medical schools had closed their doors or merged with more prestigious institutions (Sebastian, p. 165). Such a volcanic upheaval was probably both overdue and beneficial, but there were consequences that influenced the health care Americans receive today.

Without a doubt, Flexner's approach to both medical education and medical practice was elitist, with a strong bias toward specialized care. The educational changes that followed the Flexner Report started the decline of generalist practice in the U.S.—a slide that was to continue until the rise of family practice as a specialty in the late 1960s.

And so who was Abraham Flexner, who turned the great ship of American medical education? He was, the year before he began his fieldwork for the Carnegie Foundation, an unemployed former schoolmaster. His visits to medical schools were often, frankly, quite brief. Writing when he was still a medical student, Hiatt concludes that Flexner's work was "rushed and biased" and that the outcome was that "the face of the medical profession became increasingly homogeneous with respect to gender and race, its practitioners fewer but richer, its creed allopathic and interventionist, its schools dependent on grants from foundations and governments, and its reach into communities stunted" (12).

Pellagra Explained: Joseph Goldberger (1874–1929)

Pellagra, today virtually non-existent in the civilized world, might be considered a mere footnote in medical history—after all, James Lind had shown the nature of deficiency disease, scurvy—except for its impact on people in the Southeastern U.S. at the turn of the century. Reporting at the time was sketchy at best, but in 1912 the state of South Carolina reported 30,000 cases, with a 40 percent mortality rate.

Few of us have seen pellagra, a disease associated with a poor diet and poverty. The pathologic basis is a niacin deficiency that causes a troika of manifestations—diarrhea, dermatitis, and dementia. In a world just learning about germs and bacterial diseases, pellagra seemed to be one more transmissible plague. In 1914, the U.S. Congress dispatched Joseph Goldberger to Mississippi and Georgia to study the problem.

Goldberger noted that in orphanages and mental hospitals, inmates (who ate a diet based on corn products) often had pellagra, but the staff members (who ate a much more varied diet) were seldom afflicted. This was not the way a contagious disease should act at all. Goldberger postulated that diet was the cause and ran several experiments in institutions, including a state prison farm, observing persons on differing diets. He concluded that pellagra was a deficiency disease—not an infectious disease—that could be prevented and treated with a diet rich in fresh meat, vegetables, and milk.

Old beliefs die hard, and Goldberger's critics held to their belief in pellagra's contagious etiology. In 1916, Goldberger performed a dramatic demonstration. He, his wife, and several volunteer assistants held a "filth party." They swallowed pellagra scabs, inhaled dried secretions, and injected themselves with the blood of a pellagra victim. No illness occurred in the test group, convincingly demonstrating that pellagra is not a contagious disease and that there is, in fact, no "pellagra germ."

Discovery of Insulin: Frederick Banting (1891–1941) and Charles H. Best (1899–1978)

A diagnosis of diabetes mellitus was considered a death sentence until 1921, the year insulin was discovered. Working at the University of Toronto in the laboratory of physiologist J.J.R. Macleod, Frederick Banting and 22-year-old medical student Charles H. Best demonstrated that a dog became diabetic following removal of the pancreas, which contains the islets of Langerhans. (The word *insulin*, coined in 1913, comes from the Latin word *insula* [island], referring to the islets of Langerhans.) Next, they showed that injecting an extract of the islets of Langerhans could control the dog's diabetes—as long as the injections continued.

In 1922, they developed an insulin extract from the pancreas of cattle and gave the world's first insulin injection to Leonard Thompson, a diabetic teenager. The following year, insulin was made available for clinical use.

Banting and Macleod received the 1923 Nobel Prize in Physiology or Medicine. Banting was angry that Best was not honored by the Nobel Foundation and shared the cash award with him. Knighted in 1934, Banting died in 1941 when his plane crashed in Newfoundland shortly after take-off on a mission to England. Best went on to succeed Macleod as the University of Toronto professor of medicine.

Discovery of Penicillin: Alexander Fleming (1881–1955)

In 1928, Alexander Fleming, working at St. Mary's Hospital in London, returned from a vacation to find that a curious thing had occurred on a culture plate streaked with staphylococci. A colony of mold had grown on the plate, and it seemed to have blocked the growth of bacteria near it.

Instead of discarding the plate, Fleming seemed to grasp the significance of what he was seeing. He photographed the original culture plate, which was fortuitous because he attempted unsuccessfully to duplicate the phenomenon using what he thought were the same bacteria and same mold (13).

Fleming found the mold to be a member the genus *Penicillium* and named his now-legendary specimen *Penicillium notatum*. He continued experiments in vitro and later in animals; he published his results in the *British Journal of Experimental Pathology*. This written record was fortunate for Fleming's legacy, because, in the absence of human subjects, research stalled.

At Oxford, almost a decade later, Howard Florey and Ernst Chain resumed the work, borrowing a sample of Fleming's original mold colony. Animal experiments gave way to human testing. The original doses given to patients were miniscule compared to what is used today, but the staphylococci and streptococci had yet to develop "resistance," and even small doses proved effective. Research intensified as World War II began, and penicillin helped reduce the number of serious infections in injured troops.

On a personal note, I recall that in 1946, when I was about age 10, I was sick in bed with a severe cold and sore throat. Our family doctor came to the house, and he prescribed the inhalation of a new medicine—penicillin. I wondered whether my memory was correct until I found an October 11, 1948 article in *Time* magazine describing a *Journal of the American Medical Association* report of 169 patients treated with inhaled penicillin dust for colds.

Just about the time that I was inhaling penicillin dust, Fleming, Florey, and Chain were sharing the 1945 Nobel Prize in Physiology or Medicine.

Polio Vaccine: Jonas Salk (1914–1995)

Today we live in a world that is relatively free of poliomyelitis, also called infantile paralysis because of its tendency to cause permanent neurologic deficits in children as well as older individuals. Please indulge me with some more personal recollections: My mother, who grew up in upstate New York, told me of armed men at barricades in 1916, blocking entry to their town by persons fleeing an especially severe epidemic in New York City at that time. When I was young, in the 1940s, swimming in a public pool was considered putting oneself at risk for polio. When I entered medical school in 1957, there were still polio patients in iron lungs.

Working at the University of Pittsburgh, Jonas Salk devised a way to kill the poliovirus with formaldehyde and make a vaccine from the killed virus. In 1952, following in the footsteps of Edward Jenner and others, he inoculated volunteers, including his three sons, his wife, and himself. These and further experiments proved successful, and in 1955, an Associated Press dispatch read, "The Salk polio vaccine is safe, effective and potent, it was officially announced today."

Subsequently, the oral vaccine developed by Albert Sabin largely supplanted the Salk vaccine, but Salk remains identified as the one who developed the first vaccine, and in 1963, he created the Salk Institute for Biological Studies in La Jolla, California.

Human Immunodeficiency Virus Identified: Luc Montagnier (1932–) and Robert Gallo (1937–)

Senior clinicians today have lived through the evolutionary saga of HIV and AIDS, the origins of which still remain a mystery. An early hint that something new was happening was the advent of the controversial "gay bowel syndrome," a phrase coined in 1976 by a group of New York City physicians in private proctologic practice (14). As the nature of AIDS began to declare itself, having lymphadenopathy or being from the island of Haiti became reasons for suspicion.

Then in 1983, Luc Montagnier at the Pasteur Institute in Paris discovered what he called the lymphadenopathy-associated virus, or LAV. In 1984, American scientist Robert Gallo confirmed the discovery, and the virus was renamed human T lymphotropic virus type III, or HTLV-III. Considerable controversy followed the dual discoveries, including accusations that Gallo's discovery improperly involved a sample from the Pasteur Institute. In 1986, the name of the virus was changed again, this time to HIV, which is the term used today. Controversy regarding the discovery continued, however, but was more or less resolved in a meeting of no less than presidents Reagan of the U.S. and Mitterrand of France. The compromise was that there would be shared credit for the discovery of HIV.

The Twenty-First Century

Here we are in the 21st century. So far in this millennium, cloned sheep Dolly has died prematurely, Hurricane Katrina has inundated New Orleans, the U.S. has become bogged down in a war in Iraq, and the little Rover—at this writing—is still chugging around on Mars. We worry about the earth's warming, overpopulation, economic globalization, and terrorism.

So far in medicine, there has been one enduring 21st century accomplishment—the mapping of the human genome.

Human Genome Map: The International HapMap Consortium (2005)

In 2005, the International HapMap Consortium published a paper entitled "A Haplotype Map of the Human Genome" (15). The paper reports, "More than a thousand genes for rare, highly heritable 'Mendelian' disorders have been identified, in which variation in a single gene is both necessary and sufficient to cause disease." Common disorders will prove a greater challenge because in these diseases DNA variants interact with environmental factors.

As work progresses, there is hope for patients with autoimmune diseases, Alzheimer's disease, diabetes mellitus, inflammatory bowel disease, age-related macular degeneration, and many more ailments.

The release of the Human Genome Map is groundbreaking for two other reasons: First of all, is it difficult—perhaps deliberately so—to identify a single "hero." The paper lists scores of participants in the consortium (15). Second, "all data were released without restriction into the public domain" to allow the findings to be used for the greatest good of humankind.

Traits, Heroes, and Villains

Giants: Commonalities and Differences

In this chapter, I have discussed selected heroes in medical history and their accomplishments. I am sure that, in attempting to focus on the most influential contributions, I have omitted one or two of your revered medical heroes; however, your favorites may show up in the pages that follow.

Note also that we began with primitive times, when it was difficult to identify specific persons associated with advances. As if to come full circle, we end the chapter with achievements attributed to institutes and consortia—again with specific heroes hard to find in long lists of contributors.

In between the very early times and the advent of huge scientific consortia were the giants. In this section of the chapter, I wish to ponder how they were alike and how they were different.

Not All Were Physicians

We physicians are ethnocentric, each to our own specialty "tribe" and, as a group, to the community of medicine. Some, such as Rhazes and Maimonides, may be considered more philosophers than physicians. We think of Vesalius as an anatomist. Van Leeuwenhoek was a microscopist, William Morton was a dentist, Wilhelm Roentgen was a physics professor, Marie Curie was a research scientist, and William Flexner was a former schoolmaster who found employment surveying medical schools. So much for medical advances being the sole domain of physicians.

Curiosity, Persistence, and Recklessness

As a group, they seem to have had an intense need to know. Hippocrates sought relationships between nature and health; Galen, Vesalius, and Harvey conducted dissections of tissue; and Lind asked why seamen on long voyages developed scurvy. Even those who blundered into discoveries, such as Paré and Fleming, continued to work on what they had found. In many instances, curiosity was accompanied by persistence: How else can we explain the 400 microscopes built by van Leeuwenhoek, the more than 600 compounds tested by Ehrlich on his way to discovering Salvarsan, and the stubborn insistence of John Snow that the Broad Street pump—the community's water source—be taken out of service?

At other times, the curiosity gave rise to apparently reckless experimentation. Lind used seamen for his experiments, whereas Jenner gave his first vaccination to a local boy. William Morton inhaled his own ether, Wilhelm Roentgen performed the first x-ray on his wife's hand, Pierre Curie tested radium on his own skin, Joseph Goldberger and his wife consumed pellagra secretions to demonstrate that the disease was not contagious, and Jonas Salk first inoculated his sons, his wife, and himself with the new polio vaccine.

Larger Than Life

We call them giants for a reason—they cast long shadows. Imhotep was worshiped as a demigod; Maimonides, Harvey, and Jenner were physicians in royal courts. Galen promulgated a sometimes erroneous system of medicine, but it endured for centuries. Some, such as John Hunter, were notoriously irascible and short-tempered. Vesalius became angry with his colleagues and abandoned science. Semmelweis became insane.

Many received prestigious awards and prizes. Joseph Lister became Baron Lister of Lyme Regis, the first physician elevated to the British peerage. William Osler was knighted in 1911 and William Banting in 1934. There are research institutes named for Louis Pasteur and Jonas Salk.

Rejection

Throughout this chapter is a recurring theme of rejection. Early discoveries often contradicted religious beliefs. Later achievements challenged scientific dogma. Our heroes frequently encountered discouragement, ridicule, and scorn. Paré, Vesalius, and Harvey all suffered at the hands of the experts of their day. Jenner's cowpox vaccination met with early skepticism by the Royal Society, which initially refused to publish the report of his work. Semmelweis was hounded from his post in Vienna because of his insistence that the unwashed hands of clinicians might be the source of puerperal infection. Goldberger's findings initially failed to convince the experts of his time, and within our lifetime Robert Gallo has seen his work criticized on several fronts.

Writings

Our heroes wrote. Many writings are attributed to Hippocrates. Some wrote books and articles, a few of them—Galen, Rhazes, and Maimonides—authored numerous publications. Others are known for a single seminal work describing their noteworthy achievement: Vesalius' *De Humani Corporis Fabrica* (1543), Harvey's *Exercitation Anatomica du Mortu Cordis et*

Sanguinis in Animalibus (1628), Lind's *A Treatise of the Scurvy* (1753), Withering's *An Account of the Foxglove and Some of its Medical Uses* (1785), and Jenner's *An Inquiry into the Causes and Effects of Variolae Vaccinee* (1798).

In 1892, Osler single-handedly wrote a major textbook of medicine that lasted through multiple editions. Flexner's 1910 report changed medical education across a nation. Alexander Fleming might not have been revered as the man who discovered penicillin had he not written of his discovery in the *British Journal of Experimental Pathology* in 1929. If many of our giants had not written, they might never have achieved immortality and their works might have languished, awaiting later, and more literate, innovators.

Quotations and Eponyms

The giants mentioned here are remembered not only for their achievements, but also because of their recorded sayings and the ways in which many of their names have been scattered about diseases, treatments, and organs of the human body. As to quotes, Strauss' *Familiar Medical Quotations* has more than 50 quotes each attributed to Hippocrates and Osler, plus 11 quotes by Galen, 19 by Paracelsus, and 17 by Pasteur. I will present some of the most pertinent quotes in chapter 8.

Our giants have also given us many eponyms. These include hippocratic facies, Sydenham chorea, Hunterian chancre, pasteurization, Listerine, Roentgen ray, Osler-Vaquez disease, and the Salk vaccine. Look for more eponyms in chapter 5.

Longevity

Just to pick a point of reference, in 1850 in the U.S., the life expectancy of a white male at birth was 38 years; of a newborn white female, 40 years. Our heroes, in general, enjoyed relatively long lives. Hippocrates is reported to have lived to the ripe old age of 83, perhaps older; Harvey, age 79; Pasteur and Roentgen, age 77; and Osler, age 70. Pierre Curie's life was cut short by an automobile accident, Fredrick Banting's by an airplane crash. We must wonder, in passing, how many brilliant, but unheralded, persons would have contributed to medical advances if their lives had lasted longer. But we will never know.

The Villains

In this chapter, we have learned of heroes in medical history and their achievements. The other side of the coin—the dark side—represents the villains, the diseases that cause pain, disability, and premature death.

We turn to these in the next chapter.

References

1. Martí-Ibáñez F. Epilogue: to be a doctor. In: *A Prelude to Medical History*. New York, NY: MD Publications; 1961:197.
2. Reiss DY. Hippocrates—first medical writer. *Med Comm*. 1982;10:83–87.
3. Hippocrates. *Aphorisms*. Kila, MT: Kessinger Publishing Company; 2004.
4. Marcus Aurelius. *Meditations*, III. 3.
5. Cahill T. *How the Irish Saved Civilization*. New York, NY: Anchor; 1996.
6. Rosner F. The life of Moses Maimonides, a prominent medieval physician. *Einstein Q J Biol Med*. 2002;19:125–128.
7. Balint M. *The Doctor, His Patient and the Illness*. New York, NY: International Universities Press; 1957.
8. Moore W. *The Knife Man: The Extraordinary Life and Times of John Hunter: Father of Modern Surgery*. New York, NY: Broadway Books; 2005.
9. Carrell JL. *The Speckled Monster: A Historical Tale of Battling Smallpox*. New York, NY: Dutton; 2003.
10. Gawande A. On washing hands. *N Engl J Med*. 2004;350:1283–1286.
11. Osler W. *Aequanimitas with Other Addresses to Medical Students, Nurses and Practitioners of Medicine*. Philadelphia, PA: Blakiston; 1932.
12. Hiatt MD. Around the continent in 180 days: the controversial journey of Abraham Flexner. *Pharos Alpha Omega Alpha Honor Med Soc*. 1999;62:18–24.
13. Bollet AJ. Fleming's discovery of penicillin: a chance observation he couldn't repeat. *Resid Staff Physician*. July 1981:29–33.
14. Scarce M. Harbinger of plague: a bad case of gay bowel syndrome. *J Homosex*. 1997;34:1–35.
15. International HapMap Consortium. A haplotype map of the human genome. *Nature*. 2005;437:1299–1320.

2
Diseases That Changed History

In the first chapter, I discussed some of medicine's heroes and their exploits. Now we will examine the villains—the diseases that afflict humankind, the maladies that despite our best efforts seem to reemerge just when we are about to declare victory. These diseases have influenced our history, geography, culture, religion, and language.

If we were to consider only the present day and only the so-called developed world, we would list the common ailments and causes of death as cardiovascular disease, cancer, stroke, chronic lung disease, and a few others. Prevalent 21st century chronic diseases are hypertension, diabetes mellitus, degenerative joint disease (DJD), and obesity. If Galen or Thomas Sydenham could see this list, they would be shocked. In their day, the chief concern was infectious disease, which today—with the notable exception of the human immunodeficiency virus (HIV)—we keep under some measure of control with sanitation, immunizations, and antimicrobials.

Why is there a profound difference between the diseases of history and the diseases of today? Until the 20th century, the life expectancy at birth was less than 50 years. Consider that cardiovascular disease, cancer, stroke, and chronic lung disease are predominately diseases of older persons. In 1892, William Osler stated that coronary disease was "relatively rare" (Porter, p. 580). Stroke, often linked with hypertension, is uncommon in younger persons, and we awaited the 20th century to witness widespread acceptance of the daily habit of smoking one or more packs of cigarettes, now the chief cause of chronic lung disease and lung cancer. Before the introduction of insulin by Banting and Best in 1922, many people with type 1 diabetes died without having had children. Death claimed most individuals before the onset of DJD, and obesity—a disease of indulgent societal affluence—was limited to the wealthy few.

Prior to the 20th century, the chief threats to human health were the epidemic diseases—plague, smallpox, influenza, and others—that were, to use the roots of the word *epidemic*, "upon the people." They were what Martí-Ibáñez called the "collective" diseases, in contradistinction to the "individual" diseases we have today (p. 20). Most of the great epidemic diseases have always been with us. The exception is AIDS, which seems to have emerged in Sub-Saharan Africa in the 20th century.

The great epidemics are part of the fabric of the history of civilization. Bubonic plague—the Black Death—killed more than a third of Europe's population in the 14th century. At the time of the American Revolution, there was "a virulent smallpox epidemic of continental scope that claimed about 100,000 lives" (1). Today, as we ponder the threat of evolving influenza viruses, we recall tales of the worldwide influenza pandemic of 1918.

In the pages that follow, I will discuss seven infectious diseases: plague, smallpox, malaria, syphilis, measles, influenza, and tuberculosis. I am aware that I could well have added typhus, yellow fever, schistosomiasis, trypanosomiasis, and others. My choice has been guided by how much the great plagues affected the world we know today.

At the end of the chapter, I will discuss some ways in which the great plagues, and some other diseases as well, have been involved in specific events in history.

The Great Epidemics

Plague

Bubonic plague, aka the Black Death, left such an impact on humanity in late medieval times that the word *plague* has become a generic term for all widespread epidemic diseases.

First, a short review of microbiology: Bubonic plague refers to the "bubo"—an enlarged lymph node, most noticeable in the groin area. The causative organism is *Yersinia pestis*, previously named *Pasteurella pestis* in "honor" of Louis Pasteur. The classic carrier of the disease is the black rat, sometimes called the old English rat, although other rodents such as rock squirrels and prairie dogs can harbor the organism. Typically, the disease affects humans when a flea first bites an infected rat and then bites a person (Cartwright, p. 30). It can also be contracted by direct contact with the rodent. Hence, humans are most at risk for plague in settings where they live in close communion with rats or other rodents, such as in crowded city slums.

In addition to the bubonic form, there is pneumonic plague, a lung infection that, unlike the bubonic and septicemic variants, can spread from person to person by droplet infection—a much more effective means of transmission than waiting to be bitten by an infected flea—and that therefore is the most dangerous of all plague variants because it is the most readily transmissible.

I begin the tale of plague epidemics in Greece during in the fifth century BCE, the era of Hippocrates. Thucydides describes a plague that occurred during the time of the Peloponnesian War, affecting Athens in 430 BCE and continuing for three years. According to Thucydides, conditions in Athens were so dire that "men, not knowing what would happen next to them, became indifferent to every rule of religion or law" (2). Today, we are not certain whether the epidemic described by Thucydides was caused by plague, typhus, or even, as suggested by David, melioidosis (3). Whatever the cause, the fifth century plague helped set the stage for the downfall of the ancient city-state.

Plague outbreaks occurred from time to time in the centuries that followed, and in chapter 10, I will describe how these epidemics seem to have shaped the origins of Christianity.

The next epidemic of epic proportions was the so-called Plague of Justinian, occurring in the sixth century CE, during the reign of Roman emperor Justinian. The disease seems to have begun in Lower Egypt and spread to Palestine and then to the Western Roman Empire. Cartwright states that this plague "may have been the most terrible that has ever harrowed the world." At the peak of the disease, 10,000 people died daily and ships were loaded with corpses, taken to sea, and abandoned (Cartwright, p. 17). The plague, occurring at the same time as the Gothic threat from the north, certainly contributed to the fall of Rome.

Next, we move to the Black Death of 1346 to 1352. This epidemic, extending from the British Isles to Russia, killed without regard for social status, age, or gender. Millions died. Aside from the devastating mortality, the Black Death of the 14th century brought three noteworthy items.

The first is *The Decameron*, written by Italian author Giovanni Boccaccio circa 1350–1353. The collection of 100 stories is linked by the epidemic of plague that struck Florence in 1348. Ten young men and women flee from Florence and take refuge in a countryside villa for two weeks, passing the time telling stories, of which some bawdy tales of love are the best known.

The second legacy of the Black Death is the word *quarantine* (Fortuine, p. 227). The word comes from the Latin *quadraginta*, meaning 40. Venice and other Italian port cities kept arriving ships and their crews isolated for a set period. It may be that 40 days was considered to be the incubation period for infectious diseases, including plague. Alternatively, the 40 days may signify the 40 days and nights Jesus spent in the wilderness.

There was a third and grim outgrowth of the 14th century Black Death. As noted in chapter 1, the medieval era was a time of intense religiosity. Instead of seeking microorganisms as the cause of the plague (as we would do today), people sought villains or even sinners whose transgressions might be the cause of everyone's suffering. A handy target was the Jewish population, who were suspected of spreading poison to homes and wells. In Strasbourg, some 2,000 Jews were hanged. In Freiburg, they were burned. Even Ambroise Paré (1517–1564) believed that there were "plague spreaders" (Ackerknecht, p. 17). Cartwright states, "Thus the Black Death intensified the medieval Christian tradition of the scapegoat-Jew and, by causing the migration of so large a number to the east and north of Europe, is linked to the pogroms of Imperial Russia and the gas-chambers of Auschwitz" (p. 46).

In 1630, plague broke out in Venice and then spread north, eventually reaching the Tyrol and the Bavarian village of Oberammergau. Through a rigidly enforced quarantine, the residents of the small village escaped much—but not all—of the plague's devastation. In desperation, the villagers vowed that, if God would deliver them from the plague, they would present a play depicting the life and death of Jesus every decade to symbolize their gratitude. Today, you can visit the *Passionspielhaus* in the village (as I did in 1958), and once every 10 years, you can see the Oberammergau Passion Play (Major, 1936, p. 33).

The last major plague outbreak was the Great Plague of London (and Europe) that began in 1664–1665. The disease began among the poor in port areas—likely sites for cohabitation of rats and humans. It then spread to involve all of London, where the death rate reached 7,000 people per week in September 1665. Businesses closed as merchants, clergy, and physicians fled the city. Even Charles II and his court departed for Oxford. In an effort to combat the disease, fires—often scented with pepper or frankincense—were burned. Those who could afford to do so, including children, smoked tobacco as a preventive measure.

Some hold that the children's rhyme "Ring Around the Rosie" describes the plague, and specifically the Great Plague of London in 1665, although that origin is disputed. For those who believe in the plague connection, "Rosie" is the red skin rash of plague, "pocket full of posies" is scented material carried to combat disease, "ashes" may refer to the practice of burning bodies or else be an echoic allusion to coughing, and "all fall down" connotes dying.

In September 1666, much of London was destroyed in the Great Fire of London, an event that likely resulted in the death of many flea-infested rats and that was followed by a decline of the plague. As the city was rebuilt, thatched roofs were prohibited because they had proven to be a favored home for rats.

The history of plague has an interesting implication for today. In the 21st century, most of us are unlikely to suffer rat flea bites. However, *Y. pestis* is endemic among rock squirrels and other rodents in the southwestern U.S., and sporadic cases occur among campers in this area. Theoretically, today's greatest plague risk is not fleaborne disease, but droplet transmission—pneumonic plague. The development of this sort of person-to-person transmission is just what we fear today with "bird flu" and with the hemorrhagic fevers caused by the Ebola and Marburg viruses.

Smallpox

Smallpox was so named to distinguish it from the great pox—syphilis. Evidence of smallpox has been detected in the mummy of Ramses V, who died in 1157 BCE. In the 10th century CE, Rhazes provided us with the first meaningful account of the disease and distinguished between smallpox and measles. The disease smoldered endemically in various areas for hundreds of years, killing the emperors of Japan and Burma in the 16th and 17th centuries, until being eradicated (we hope) in the latter half of the 20th century.

Today, we think of smallpox as a historical curiosity. Within my lifetime, however, it was a reality. As a child and later as I prepared for international travel, I was vaccinated several times, as were both of my children. As a young practicing physician, I administered vaccinations to hundreds of patients, always mindful that I should not vaccinate patients who personally had or who might expose persons with eczema or immunodeficiency.

One memorable encounter with smallpox occurred in 1963, when I was serving as a staff physician at the U.S. Public Health Service (USPHS) Hospital at Norfolk, Virginia. At the time, the USPHS provided health care for a variety of constituencies, including merchant seaman employed on vessels registered both in the U.S. and abroad. One day we received a message that a ship flying a Liberian flag was headed our way with a seaman with smallpox aboard. In 1963, this was a perfectly possible scenario. Hastily, we vaccinated all hospital employees whose vaccination status was not current. We evacuated a wing of the hospital to serve as an isolation unit and called for volunteers—with up-to-date vaccinations—to serve there.

Then one courageous young doctor stepped forward to remove the infected patient from the merchant ship at sea. He set out early in the morning. We held our breath and stocked our hospital's newly created isolation wing. Finally, just after supper, our doctor returned from the port in an ambulance, bringing with him the infected patient, who had a clear-cut case of adult chickenpox.

A dramatic historical impact of smallpox occurred at the time of the Spanish conquest of Mexico. In 1519, Hernán Cortés and several hundred adventurers landed in Mexico, bringing with them horses, dogs, armor, gunpowder, and the smallpox virus. The ruling Aztecs and their emperor Montezuma learned of the landing and kept track of the Spaniards' progress. Cortés and the conquistadors advanced on the capital city, Tenochtitlan, aided by local tribes fed up with the Aztec rule and by a legend that a winged god, Quetzalcoatl, would arrive on the east wind and subdue the Aztec rulers. The Aztecs saw Cortés, arriving on sailing ships from the east, as the arriving Quetzalcoatl, affording him mythical power in their eyes.

The conquistadors, with superior firepower, captured Tenochtitlan (now Mexico City). But in June 1520 the Aztecs mounted a revolt and drove the Spaniards from the city. On the night the Aztecs reconquered their city, a smallpox epidemic began. The results were fearful, especially because the Aztecs saw that the Spaniards, largely immune because of exposure in Europe, were spared by the smallpox epidemic.

In April 1521, Cortés returned with reinforcements, laying siege and eventually taking the city in August 1521. The victorious Spaniards found buildings filled with bodies covered with pox. It is fair to say that the conquest of Mexico—with a small force toppling an empire—can be ascribed to a convenient legend and superior firepower, but also to a smallpox epidemic inadvertently initiated by the invaders.

By the end of the conquest of Mexico and the New World, more than a third of all the indigenous people had died of smallpox. The surviving native persons were subjugated by the Spaniards. Their culture and historical records were destroyed, to be replaced by a new language and a new religion.

Smallpox continued to play a role in American history. In Pennsylvania in 1763, the British fought a battle against tribes of Native Americans led by chief Pontiac. British officer Sir Jeffery Amherst, aware of the Indians' susceptibility to smallpox, is reported to have sent them blankets infected with the disease. History is unclear whether this actually occurred, but in the months that followed smallpox was reported in several tribes in the area.

Smallpox was endemic in the colonies at the time of the American Revolution. General George Washington, by coincidence, had apparently acquired immunity to smallpox during a time spent in Barbados in his youth. Washington, however, recognized the value of maintaining the health of his troops and ordered arm-to-arm inoculation of his troops. In his biography of Washington, Ellis calls this "the most important strategic decision of his military career" (1).

Smallpox was eventually conquered by "disease control" measures. There is still no effective antimicrobial agent. As the incidence declined with mass vaccinations, public health officials adopted a policy of identifying and then controlling (isolating) infected individuals, continuing this practice over and over in developing countries until October 26, 1977. On that day, a 23-year-old cook, Ali Maow Malin, in the town of Marka, in Somalia, was designated by the World Health Organization (WHO) as having the world's last naturally occurring case of smallpox.

Sadly, I must qualify the previous sentence with the phrase "naturally occurring" because, in our infinite wisdom, we have maintained laboratory samples of the smallpox virus, causing the legitimate concern today that these virus samples might be acquired and used by terrorists.

Malaria

Malaria, the word coming from the Italian *mal* (bad) and *aria* (air), was once thought to be caused by toxic vapors coming from swamps. Today, we know that it is not the "bad air" from damp areas but the mosquito vectors likely to be found there. In fact, because the *Anopheles* mosquitoes that carry *Plasmodia* seldom have a suitable habitat in cities, malaria is generally a disease of jungles, swamps, and forests.

Malaria has exerted a selective, darwinian influence on the incidence of genetic diseases. One manifestation of this impact is in relation to sickle cell anemia. An autosomal dominant inherited disease, sickle cell anemia is caused by a mutation of the HBB gene related to a hemoglobin subunit. The abnormality affects some 2.5 million people in the U.S., about 8%–10% of the country's African-American population, and also occurs in some non-black persons. A minority of those affected are homozygous for the sickle cell gene; these people have sickle cell disease and often die young. Most are heterozygous and have the sickle cell trait; these people have significant resistance to malaria. A similar protection occurs in people with glucose-6-phosphate dehydrogenase deficiency who are susceptible to favism.

What appear to be malarial epidemics have occurred throughout history. Evidence is found in artifacts from ancient China, Egypt, Babylon, Palestine, and India. Malaria is discussed in several of the works of Hippocrates. The disease has been implicated as a cause of the decline of both ancient Greece and Rome. Malaria was recorded in farm areas on the outskirts of Rome in the first century BCE and persisted for five centuries. Cartwright states, "Possibly malaria, rather than decadent luxury imported from the East, accounted for the slackness of spirit which characterized the later years of Rome" (p. 11).

A key chapter in the story of malaria was written in Central America with the construction of the Panama Canal. The first attempt to build a waterway was by the French in the mid-1880s. In this effort, some 5,000 workmen died—most succumbing to malaria and yellow fever. When the U.S. later acquired the right to construct a canal, workmen found that the area was awash with manmade mosquito breeding grounds. The French had used moats and pools of water to protect themselves from umbrella ants, thereby creating veritable mosquito incubators. The Americans set about removing or applying insecticides to the pools of still water and using mosquito-proof netting both for protection and to isolate infected individuals.

Eventually, the Panama Canal opened in 1914, a triumph for both American engineering and public health measures. What's more, as stated by Porter (p. 471), "This parasitological model opened up an astonishing new vision of disease etiology."

A key player in the malaria drama was Scottish physician Sir Ronald Ross (1857–1932), who showed that the *Anopheles* mosquito carries the malaria parasite and who was awarded the 1902 Nobel Prize in Physiology or Medicine. Ross, whose passion was writing poetry, recorded his finding in verse:

> I know this little thing
> A myriad of men will save
> O Death, where is thy sting?
> Thy victory, O Grave?

The reader may recognize the last two lines as borrowed from the Bible: 1 Corinthians 15:55.

I wish I could report that the glory days of malaria ended with the identification of the parasite and its vector, but the story continues. The disease was present in the U.S. as late as the 19th century, accentuated at that time by the great westward migration and the Civil War. The armies of World War I experienced malaria, and Ackerknecht (p. 94) states that, "In World War II malaria was the main medical problem of military forces engaged in the Pacific as well as in the Mediterranean areas."

Today, more than 300 million people worldwide are infected with the malaria parasite, and up to 1–3 million die annually. The disease is most prevalent in Sub-Saharan Africa, and most deaths are in children under age 5. Statistics are vague, at best, because most malaria cases and most deaths are undocumented.

Syphilis

Syphilis, aka lues, is a favorite of medical historians for several reasons. The word *syphilis* evokes a literary image. It is a disease with truly protean manifestations, and Osler once stated, "The physician who knows syphilis knows medicine." The disease has no respect for social class and has infected hundreds of well-known persons. And although its epidemiologic origins are debated even today, its early migration across national boundaries can be traced with reasonable certainty.

A sexually transmitted disease, syphilis is caused by a spirochetal bacterium, *Treponema pallidum*. With some exceptions such as congenital syphilis, the disease is spread from human to human by intimate sexual contact. Irish surgeon Abraham Colles (1773–1843), namesake of the Colles fracture, discussed the transmission of syphilis: "I may be told by some that men may contract syphilis by sitting in a public privy; to this I can only answer that I have never witnessed a single instance; nor did the late Mr. Obre, who had been for many years most extensively engaged in treating the venereal disease; for on asking him if he believed that the disease was propagated in this manner, he shrewdly answered that it sometimes was the manner in which married men contracted it, but unmarried men never caught it in this manner" (Strauss, p. 651).

In the late 1950s, an aging patriarch who had developed one of the early serologic tests for the disease gave my medical school lecture on the topic. This venerated physician (whose name I will not divulge) proclaimed, "Whenever a young man tells me that he contracted the disease from a public toilet, I tell him, 'That is an awful place to take a woman.'" I suspect that this story would be considered inappropriate in a medical school classroom today, but it does make a point.

What about the word *syphilis*? Sipylus, sometimes spelled Siphylus, was first the hero of a love poem entitled *Metamorphoses*, written by the Roman poet Ovid in the first century CE (Gershen, p. 100). Later, in 1530, Veronese physician Girolamo Fracastorius (1483–1553) used the name in a poem entitled *Syphilis, sive Morbus Gallicus* (Syphilis, or the French Disease), thereby beginning the tradition of blaming others for the infection. In Fracastorius' poem, the sad hero was punished for offending the sun god Apollo: "And first among them all, Syphilus, who had established the worship of the King with blood-sacrifices, and raised altars to him among the mountains, manifested the foul sores in his own body. . . . And from him, first to suffer it, the disease took its name and was called syphilis by the native race" (4).

In fact, we are not at all sure who the first person to suffer the disease was, and scholars debate various theories as to its origin. A favorite, but often challenged, story is the Columbian theory that the disease was contracted from the natives of Hispaniola in 1492 by the sailors with Christopher Columbus and returned with them to Spain. Spaniards then carried the infection to Italy, where they infected some local girls, who in turn infected troops of French King Charles VIII as they laid siege to Naples in 1495. It is speculated that wily Neapolitans may have purposely sent infected prostitutes to carry the disease to the French invaders (Haubrich, p. 237).

Whatever happened in Naples, the French troops became carriers and they seem to have liberally shared the disease across Europe. Thus, we better understand Fracastorius' 1530 subtitle, "the French disease." In fact, in various settings, syphilis has been called the French disease, the Italian disease, the Neapolitan disease, and the Spanish disease. The Russians have called it the Polish disease, the Japanese have called it the Chinese pleasure disease, and the Arabs have called it the Christian disease. The French called it the great pox, to differentiate it from smallpox.

Of course, the Columbian theory raises the question as to the origin of the disease in the New World. In this regard, Ackerknecht writes, "A few South American scientists have attempted to trace the disease back even further and assumed that syphilis had originally been a disease of the South American llamas and that these llamas had infected the natives who had a great affection for these animals" (p. 118).

Pre-Columbian theory skeptics hold that there is evidence of syphilis in the Bible, with the sins of the father visited unto future generations (Exodus 20:5). Other scholars believe that some writings attributed to Hippocrates describe the symptoms and signs of syphilis. Yet another intriguing theory holds that syphilis is a form of the *Treponemal* disease yaws which evolved when introduced into a new ecological setting. The epidemiologic chronology of syphilis is still debated.

Those who contracted syphilis in the centuries following Columbus and Fracastorius were in august company. Some believe that the disease afflicted not just his sailors but Columbus himself. French King Charles VIII died of syphilis in 1498 at age 28 and was succeeded on the throne by several syphilitic rulers. The disease was not confined to continental Europe. It was contracted by English King Henry VIII and five of his wives.

Some believe that the great pox that infected many in Europe in the 16th century was a more virulent disease than we see today. After all, according to Bollet, one third of the inhabitants of Paris were infected at that time, and Erasmus (1466–1536) stated that a nobleman who had not yet had syphilis was "*ignobilis et rusticanus*" (4). In 1957, on my first trip to France, my host shared the aphorism that, "No Frenchman can live to the age of 60 without getting syphilis, cirrhosis, or the Legion of Honor."

There is reasonable evidence that the following persons had syphilis or else believed they were infected with the disease (5,6):

> Meriwether Lewis (of Lewis and Clark fame)
> Franz Schubert
> Lord Randolph Churchill (father of Sir Winston Churchill)
> Guy de Maupassant
> Vincent van Gogh
> Paul Gauguin
> Mary Todd Lincoln
> Henri de Toulouse-Lautrec
> Vladimir Lenin
> Al Capone
> Howard Hughes

In 1877, Guy de Maupassant seemed to take some pride in his affliction: "I've got the pox! At last! Not the contemptible clap . . . no, no—the great pox, the one Francis I died of. The majestic pox . . . and I'm proud of it, by thunder. I don't have to worry about catching it anymore, and I screw the street whores and trollops, and afterwards I say to them, 'I've got the pox.'" (Porter, p. 451).

Having contracted syphilis in his youth, Al Capone eventually reached the stage of neurosyphilis, which caused confusion and bizarre behavior during his time in Alcatraz.

There is another list of persons who may have had syphilis, but we are not quite sure whether all listed were infected. If they did, however, some familiar historical events may be explained. Some of the persons on this list are (5,6):

> Queen Elizabeth I
> Ivan the Terrible, of Russia
> Wolfgang Amadeus Mozart
> Napoleon Bonaparte
> Ludwig van Beethoven
> Edgar Allan Poe
> Charles Darwin
> Abraham Lincoln
> Fyodor Dostoevsky
> Edouard Manet

Oscar Wilde
Joseph Stalin
James Joyce
Adolf Hitler
Henry Miller
Idi Amin

As a historical note indicating the significance of syphilis in medicine at the time, the American Board of Dermatology and Syphilology was incorporated in 1932 and was not changed to the American Board of Dermatology until 1955.

With the widespread availability of penicillin following World War II, the eradication of syphilis became theoretically possible, just as we have eliminated naturally occurring smallpox from the world. But with human inclinations and behavior being what they are, as of today the eradication of syphilis must remain a much-desired possibility.

Influenza

Most of us have experienced "the flu," a syndrome of fever, overwhelming malaise, headache, and muscle aches. Typically, the symptoms last a few days and then we begin to recover. You and I generally achieve our pre-flu healthy status within a week or two of the onset of symptoms. We consider influenza an unpleasant temporary illness and little more. The story seems to have been different in past centuries.

According to Ackerknecht, "The ancients never gave an unequivocal description of the disease" (p. 74). The name *influenza* comes directly from a Latin word *influencia*, referring to "influential coeli," or heavenly influence. The word first appears in the *History of Florence*, written by Buoninsegni in 1580, in reference to the 1357 epidemic (Garrison, p. 187). The term was adopted into the English language in the 18th century; the French preferred the term *grippe* (Garrison, p. 404).

Over the centuries, influenza tended to occur in pandemics, although a few of the early descriptions of "sweating sickness" were really something else. As with syphilis, there is an ethnocentric tendency to blame the illness on "them." Hence, in Italy, it was called "the German disease," in Germany "the Russian pestilence," and in Russia "the Chinese disease" (Haubrich, p. 121). In the U.S., we have experienced the Asian flu and Hong Kong flu. Nor have other living things escaped blame. Witness the terms "swine flu" and "bird flu."

The epic tale of influenza describes what happened in 1918 and afterward. As influenza spread worldwide, it claimed the lives of more than 25 million people, more than three times the number of individuals killed in World War I. Porter describes the 1918 influenza episode as "the most mobile and lethal pandemic the world has ever seen." As one example, Porter (p. 483) describes what happened in Boston: influenza struck 1 person in 10, and those afflicted had a 60 percent rate of mortality. Not only was the disease lethal, some survivors were afflicted with encephalitis lethargica, an inflammation of the spinal cord and brain.

Encephalitis lethargica, also called von Economo disease in honor of Austrian neurologist Constantin F. von Economo (1876–1931), seems to have been a one-of-a-kind encephalitis. It caused severe somnolence and often ophthalmoplegia, and many victims suffered postencephalitic parkinsonism. During my time in the USPHS (1961–1964), I encountered several elderly individuals with parkinsonism that they could trace to the 1918 influenza epidemic.

Influenza probably played a significant—perhaps decisive—role in the First World War. By the spring of 1918, the German army had more than 1 million battle-hardened troops on the Western Front. French and British troops were outnumbered and desperate. American forces had not yet arrived in sufficient numbers to turn the tide. By May, the Germans were within artillery range of Paris. For them, victory seemed to require only a swift and decisive attack.

But the attack did not come. The German commander, General Erich Ludendorff, paused, and during this interval, more American troops arrived and the Allies gathered strength. The eventual German offensive failed, and the tide of the war changed.

Why did the German army choose to rest within sight of Paris? Yes, the German army had driven west very rapidly and needed to secure their supply lines. History tells us that food for the German troops was in short supply. However, Ludendorff himself attributed the delay and eventual defeat to his troops' having influenza, which the Germans called the *Blitzkatarrh* (7). At one time, more than 2,000 troops in each German division were incapacitated with influenza (Oldstone, p. 173).

Over the years, influenza has revisited us, causing annual outbreaks of greater or lesser severity. Some outbreaks have had curious features. The 1976 swine flu epidemic caused some persons to have Guillain-Barré syndrome, a phenomenon that I noted in three patients in my rural practice at that time. Antigenic drift of the virus' genetic material has forced us to modify our influenza vaccine each year.

As I write, we are all concerned about the emergence of the so-called bird flu. The history of influenza is still being written.

Tuberculosis

When we think of tuberculosis (TB), we think of Mimì, the tragic heroine of Puccini's opera *La Bohème*; John "Doc" Holliday, the gunslinging dentist who fought beside the Earp brothers at the O.K. Corral, and the sanitorium in Thomas Mann's *The Magic Mountain*. TB has always had a mystique, which would be engaging if the disease were not so debilitating and so often fatal.

We have found evidence of TB in mummies from ancient Egypt and in the bones of early Native Americans. Our fifth century BCE hero, Hippocrates, described TB, noting that it was the most prevalent disease of his time. In the early 1800s, a quarter of all deaths in England were caused by TB; a century later, at the end of World War I, TB caused one sixth of all deaths in France. With the development of antitubercular drugs during the 1900s, the world dared to hope that the disease could be eradicated, but the emergence of drug-resistant strains has led to a resurgence of TB, prompting the WHO to declare a global health emergency in 1993.

When we think of deaths due to TB, we think of adults. Shryock (p. 96) offers some insight into why as he writes of life in 18th century America: "The dangerous decades in the life span were the first, second, and the fourth—so far as total deaths were concerned. In other words, individuals who survived the tenth year had relatively good prospects until they reached the twenties, when tuberculosis and other respiratory diseases began to take their toll."

TB has been known by many names. It was called *phthisis* by ancient Greeks, and later in England it was "the King's evil" because of the belief that cures could follow the king's touch. The term "white plague" connotes the victims' pallor, and "miliary tuberculosis" alludes to a radiologic appearance that is similar to millet seeds. Scrofula describes TB of the cervical lymphatics, *lupus vulgaris* (literally, the common wolf) is a term for disease of the skin, and *tabes mesenterica* is TB of the abdomen. A special type of skin TB is "prosector's wart," indicating that pathologists and anatomists occasionally contracted the disease from contaminated cadavers.

Mycobacterium tuberculosis was described in 1882 by Robert Koch (1843–1910), earning him a 1905 Nobel Prize. Koch, however, subsequently tarnished his image with a misadventure that I describe in chapter 11.

Fundamentally, TB was and is a disease of crowded conditions, often the case in urban settings, notably in neighborhoods populated by the poor. But because the illnesses of poor individuals are often not recorded, the roster of famous TB victims is a list of history's rich, famous, and talented. Here are some of the tubercular notables (although not all died of the disease) (8):

John Keats
Albert Camus
Frédéric Chopin
Paul Gauguin
Franz Kafka
Washington Irving
Edgar Allan Poe
René Laennec (French physician)
Anton Chekhov
Ulysses S. Grant
Sarah Bernhardt

Simón Bolívar
Jimmie Rodgers (American musician)
Eleanor Roosevelt
Nelson Mandela

TB is mentioned often in literature and is found in the works of Sir Arthur Conan Doyle (himself a physician), Fyodor Dostoevsky, Charles Dickens, Kurt Vonnegut, John le Carré, Sylvia Plath, and Mark Helprin. Writing in his diary, Thomas Moore (1779–1852) described Lord Byron after his illness at Petras: the Romantic poet, regarding his image in a mirror, reflected, "I look pale; I should like to die of consumption. Why? Because the ladies would all say, 'Look at that poor Byron, how interesting he looks in dying.'" (Strauss, p. 643). Writing of 18th and 19th century America, Shryock (p. 120) comments, "Contemporary novels, plays, and operas were so given to sweet-sad musings [about the manifestations of TB] that consumption may be said to have made a morbid contribution to art and letters."

American physician E.L. Kendig writes of his personal experience with the disease: "When, in 1942, I was called for active military duty, my chest roentgenogram revealed changes compatible with active pulmonary disease. I became a patient at the Trudeau Sanitorium." He goes on to tell of care he receives and how, at the time he wrote the article, he was age 85 and still playing tennis (9).

In the days before World War II, roentgenography was not as advanced as it is today. My father, born in 1899 and raised on a farm in Northwest Ohio (pay attention to this clue), had been a reserve officer in World War I. In the summer of 1941, he rejoined the military in the buildup that preceded the U.S. entry into World War II in December of that year. He was sent to a U.S. Army training camp in Biloxi, Mississippi, and later assigned to active duty, when one day in October 1941, the commanding officer called Dad into his office. "Captain Taylor," he said, "I am sorry to inform you that you have advanced pulmonary tuberculosis. You are hereby medically discharged from the Army. I am very sorry to have to give you this bad news."

And so, a few months before Pearl Harbor, my father was sent home with his medical discharge. He worked until age 65 and then enjoyed 31 years of active retirement until he died after a fall at age 96. What was my father's illness in 1941? In my opinion, offered in the grand tradition of retrospective diagnosis, Dad had histoplasmosis, which he contracted during his days as a farm boy working in chicken coops and from which he made a spontaneous and full recovery.

The Trudeau Sanitorium where Dr. Kendig was treated in 1942 is an important chapter in the history of TB. Edward L. Trudeau, a physician who himself developed TB, moved to the Adirondack Mountain community of Saranac Lake, New York, and found that he returned to good health. There, in 1885, Trudeau built a sanitorium that emphasized rest, relaxation, and fresh air. Many patients used the "cure chair"—a cross between a hospital bed and chaise lounge. Also, some patients were treated by artificial pneumothorax to collapse infected lung tissue, a popular remedy of the time. By the mid-20th century, the name Saranac Lake had become synonymous with TB treatment.

This brings me to my own personal story. In the summer of 1954, at age 18, I accepted a job at a summer camp on the shores of Upper Saranac Lake, very near to Saranac Lake Village. To my parents, this meant that I was going to the country's epicenter of TB! My family feared for my health and worried all summer while I enjoyed the camp activities and the clean mountain air. I did not contract TB, heard virtually nothing about the sanitorium while I was there, and later learned that 1954 was the year in which the sanitorium closed, subsequently to become the home of the American Management Association.

Today, we risk complacency with TB, while each year the case rates rise when they should be falling. The reasons include drug-resistant organisms, the increasing number of immunocompromised individuals in the community, and uncontrolled immigration to the U.S. In the words of Dr. Kendig, "And remember, the great white plague is back" (9).

Selected Short Tales of Times When Disease Influenced History

So far in this chapter, I have discussed some of the major epidemics that have plagued humankind since ancient times, recurring from time to time to influence what we read in history books. This section describes some specific instances in which disease shaped events, beginning in medieval times and ending with decisions at the end of World War II.

Black Death: One Positive Outcome

Above, I discussed plague, which ravaged Europe in the 14th century. At that time, England was hard hit, especially since the disease incidence was rising just when manpower was needed to tend crops in the fields. Also at that time, England and France were engaged in one of their seemingly perpetual wars.

Because of the deaths of so many young men on both sides of the channel and the need for the able-bodied survivors to cultivate the crops, France and England entered into a truce on May 2, 1349. Hostilities did not resume until September 1355, as the plague was waning in both counties (Cartwright, p. 41).

Yellow Fever and Slavery in America

The yellow fever virus was one factor actually increasing the importation of African slaves following the Spanish conquest of the New World in the 16th century. The virus came to America from Africa aboard ships bringing trade goods and often slaves. Native Americans, lacking prior exposure to the disease, died in large numbers, leaving a shortage of workers in the fields and mines. In contrast, the imported African slaves seemed to have relative resistance to the disease.

The landlords and mine owners did what they considered the only logical thing: They increased the number of imported African slaves, thereby expanding the slave trade in the New World (Oldstone, p. 4).

Scurvy and Captain Cook

In chapter 1, I told of James Lind and his 1753 publication of *A Treatise of the Scurvy*. Despite Lind's research, which included several types of therapy in addition to citrus, the British Admiralty seemed to yawn at his findings.

One person, however, did not. Captain James Cook, on his historic 1772–1775 voyage to the South Pacific, provided each of his seamen with a ration of lemon juice. On this trip, Cook and his ship HMS *Resolution* visited Tahiti, Easter Island, and the Friendly Islands. The *Resolution* remained free of scurvy during the three-year voyage, undoubtedly contributing to the success of the endeavor. However, as reported by Inglis (p. 115), the Admiralty "remained unimpressed" with antiscorbutic prophylaxis.

Syphilis and Captain Cook

On his third and final voyage, Captain Cook commanded the HMS *Discovery*. During the years 1776–1779, this ship and her crew visited the Hawaiian Islands and the west coast of North America. The Hawaiian Islands had escaped the attention of seagoing explorers until 1778, when Cook and his crew landed there, becoming the first Europeans to do so. They brought with them syphilis, previously unknown in the Pacific Islands.

Over the next hundred years, syphilis, smallpox, measles, and other diseases carried by visiting Europeans resulted in the deaths of up to 90 percent of the native Hawaiian population (Porter, p. 466).

As an ironic historic note, Cook returned to Hawaii in 1779. While docked in the harbor of Kealakekua Bay, some Hawaiians made off with one of the ship's small boats. Cook and the crew could not ignore the theft and sought to retrieve the boat by taking hostage Hawaiian Chief Kalaniopu'u. A clash ensued, shots were fired, and Captain Cook was stabbed and clubbed to death by the angry Hawaiians—who unknowingly achieved some measure of revenge for the syphilitic epidemic inflicted upon them.

Typhus and Napoleon's Russian Campaign

I have always believed that, in the 1812 Russian campaign, Napoleon Bonaparte's army was defeated on its retreat from Moscow. Cartwright (pp. 90–112) holds that this statement does not tell the whole story. The seeds of defeat were actually sown in the outbound journey. Typhus, plus hunger and war wounds, played important roles during the eastbound march, the battles themselves, and the sad trip home.

In June 1812, Napoleon left East Germany with an army of more than a half million men, double the number of troops in the Russian armies. As they marched toward Russia, they raced ahead of their supplies. Food and water shortages became serious problems for the huge army. On their way east through Poland, the French army contracted typhus, which would beleaguer them until their return to France.

By July 1812, there had been more than 80,000 typhus deaths among the soldiers, with 300 miles yet to travel to Moscow. By the end of July, Napoleon's officers reported to him that illness and desertion had reduced his effective fighting force by half. By the time Napoleon reached Moscow, his army numbered less than 100,000 able-bodied men. Napoleon conquered Moscow, by then a devastated city, with no storehouses of food to feed his army. Some French reinforcements arrived, but Napoleon's troops still faced continuing typhus, starvation, and the prospect of the fierce Russian winter.

On October 19, 1812, some 95,000 bedraggled troops began the trip home. As they marched west, they were harassed by Russian troops and suffered the effects of food shortages, the winter snows, and the ever-present typhus. Men died and were left along the road. In December 1812, the original army of a half million men was reduced to about 25,000; most of these did not live to return to France.

Perhaps without the typhus deaths, Napoleon's Russian campaign might have survived the food shortages, the battles, and the snow. We can only wonder what might have happened if typhus had not infected the eastward-bound French troops.

Measles and Its Travels

As if the South Sea epidemics introduced by Captain Cook and other sailors who followed were not enough, another plague arrived just over a century later. In October 1874, England annexed the Fiji Islands. Early the following year, the HMS *Dido* docked at the islands, and her crew brought measles (Oldstone, p. 73).

When I was young, we considered measles—along with mumps and chickenpox—to be one of the "usual childhood diseases," conveniently abbreviated on medical histories as UCD. These diseases were usually minor childhood events, something to have and "get over" and then be blessed with lifelong immunity.

But when the measles virus is introduced into an immunologically naïve population, the results can be disastrous. Virtually everyone in the Fijian population contracted the disease. Affected persons sought relief from high fevers by immersion in the ocean. Some of those who contracted the disease survived to enjoy future immunity. Eventually, up to 40 percent of the native Fijian population died. From Fiji, the disease spread from island to island in the South Pacific, in each instance recreating the picture of suffering and death.

Hemophilia, Queen Victoria, and the Russian Monarchy

Hemophilia A is well known as the curse of the Romanov family. The disease is a sex-linked genetic disorder involving a single gene on the X chromosome. Women with this genetic heritage rarely develop hemophilia but can pass the disease on to their sons. How did hemophilia come to afflict the royal family of tzarist Russia?

In Europe, it has long been the custom for royal families to marry their offspring to other royals. This forms handy alliances and presumably may forestall future armed conflicts. One such union was the 1894 marriage of Nicholas II, Tzar and Emperor of All the Russias, and Alix, aka Alexandra, the granddaughter of Victoria, Queen of Great Britain. Alexandra unwittingly introduced the hemophilia gene into the Romanov line.

Nicholas and Alexandra had one son, Alexei (born August 12, 1904), who developed hemophilia. Repeated bleeding episodes nearly caused Alexei's death on several occasions. In desperation, the frightened parents invited into their home the mystic Grigori Rasputin, sometimes called the "evil monk," who perhaps used hypnosis to calm the frightened child during bleeding episodes. Before long, Rasputin's power in the royal household increased, causing concern and resentment in the *Duma* and among the public.

It is logical to speculate that Nicholas II was distracted from his royal duties by his concern for his son while his subjects feared the influence of Rasputin, factors that helped set the stage for the Russian Revolution of 1917, which ended the house of Romanov.

In the end, Rasputin was murdered in 1916 in a very thorough manner. He was first poisoned, then shot, then beaten, and eventually drowned in a river. The Romanov family was massacred in July 1918. In 1981, the Russian Orthodox Church canonized Nicholas II and his family as saints.

Hypertension, Heart Failure, and the Grand Alliance

The last story in this section highlights an important concept: As we look at the great plagues that have occurred over past millennia, it is easy to believe that all the diseases that have shaped civilization were those that affected populations or even families. Some diseases that affect history are "individual diseases."

As the impact of epidemics has waned (at least for now), the diseases of aging have commanded our attention, and illness affecting a single key individual—notably a political leader—can also have a profound effect on entire nations. In world history, pivotal episodes occur when degenerative disease strikes an influential leader at just the wrong time. Let us look at one such instance.

As World War II ended, the leaders of the Allied powers—Winston Churchill, Joseph Stalin, and Franklin D. Roosevelt—met at Yalta in February 1945 to plan what would happen to the various warring countries in the years to follow. Although not all agree, many hold that Roosevelt was mentally impaired at the meeting and that he made errors in negotiation that he would not have made had he been in good health.

We know now that Roosevelt had chronic hypertension, in addition to suffering the residual effects of polio. By March 1944, a Bethesda Naval Hospital examination revealed that he had hypertension, heart disease, left ventricular failure, and bronchitis. Remarkably, no one seems to have told the president of his failing health.

By the time of the Yalta Conference, his blood pressure had climbed to alarming heights. Recall that, in 1945, we lacked the panoply of antihypertensive medications we have today. Roosevelt had lost weight and appeared weak. We believe that he had severe hypertensive cardiac failure with cachexia and, notably, hypoxemia with impaired cerebral oxygenation.

At the conference, Roosevelt failed to assert himself in his dealings with the robust and aggressive Stalin. Thus, the agreement reached allowed Stalin later to seize Manchuria, gain control of Poland, and establish buffer states to protect his homeland.

A month later, Roosevelt's blood pressure was 240/180 mm Hg. Still, his physicians did not worry the president with details of his illness, perhaps because there was little they could do for him.

On April 12, 1945, just two months after the Yalta Conference, Roosevelt died of a cerebral hemorrhage. His personal physician reported that the fatal stroke had come "out of the clear sky" (10).

For readers who wish to learn more about what happens when disease affects influential persons, I recommend the book by Robins and Post, *When Illness Strikes the Leader: The Dilemma of the Captive King* (11).

References

1. Ellis JJ. *His Excellency: George Washington*. New York, NY: Knopf; 2005:86–87.
2. Thucydides. *History of the Peloponnesian War*. Warner R, trans. New York, NY: Penguin Books; 1954.

3. David EM. "The good and the bad dying indiscriminately": the Athenian plague reconsidered. *Pharos Alpha Omega Alpha Honor Med Soc*. 2000;63:4–7.
4. Bollet AJ. Syphilis: the French disease? *Med Times*. 1982;110:25–29.
5. Hayden D. *Pox: Genius, Madness, and the Mysteries of Syphilis*. New York, NY: Basic Books; 2003.
6. List of well-known and suspected syphilis patients. Available at: http://en.wikipedia.org/wiki/Syphilis#Well-known_and_suspected_syphilis_patients. Accessed May 4, 2007.
7. Bollet AJ. Wilson and the influenza epidemic of 1918. *Med Times*. 1983;111:100–107.
8. List of tuberculosis victims. Available at: http://en.wikipedia.org/wiki/List_of_tuberculosis_victims/. Accessed May 4, 2007.
9. Kendig EL Jr. The great white plague: a personal memoir. *Pharos Alpha Omega Alpha Honor Med Soc*. 1996;59:8–10.
10. Hamdy RC. Hypertension: a turning point in the history of medicine . . . and mankind. *South Med J*. 2001;94:1045–1047.
11. Robins RS, Post JM. *When Illness Strikes the Leader: The Dilemma of the Captive King*. New Haven, CT: Yale University Press; 1995.

3
Drugs and Other Remedies

In the first two chapters, I discussed some of medicine's heroes and their exploits and several of the diseases that have affected humans and our world. There is another important collection of tales; these are about the drugs and other remedies that physicians and scientists have developed to combat the illnesses we all suffer. Some drugs, such as quinine, originally came from botanicals; ergot and penicillin were discovered in fungi; conjugated equine estrogens (Premarin) was extracted from horse urine; and one of the compounds we use today—ammonia—was first derived from camel dung. Drawing laboratory notes from a hat decided the patent rights of isoniazid. In this third chapter, I discuss six historically noteworthy compounds—ranging from the opium derivatives to penicillin. As a bonus, I will share some short stories about other familiar medications such as nitrogen mustard, warfarin, and nystatin.

Opium and Its Derivatives

Over the millennia, opium and its derivatives have been both a blessing and a curse for humankind. These drugs have eased the pain of traumatic wounds, surgery, and heart attacks and can also help control dysentery and relieve the dyspnea of heart failure. But on the dark side, their addictive properties have ruined many lives.

We can trace the use of opium to Egypt in the second millennium BCE. Medieval Persian physician and scientist Avicenna (980–1037) called it the "most powerful of the stupefacients" (Porter, p. 194). Paracelsus (1493–1541) was an enthusiastic proponent of opium therapy. In the next century, Thomas Sydenham (1624–1689) wrote, "Among the remedies which it has pleased Almighty God to give to man to relieve his sufferings, none is so universal and so efficacious as opium" (Fortuine, p. 312).

In the 18th century, Scottish physician John Cheyne (for whom Cheyne-Stokes respiration is named) continued to praise opium, by then widely used to relieve pain, reduce fever, and combat diarrhea. Cheyne wrote,

"Providence has been kind and gracious to us beyond all Expression in furnishing us with a certain Relief, if not a Remedy, even to our most intense Pains and extreme Miseries" (Porter, p. 269).

In 1806 in Germany, F.W.A. Sertürner isolated morphine, which Fortuine describes as "one of the earliest chemically pure medications derived from plants to become available to physicians" (p. 315). In 1832, Pierre Jean Robiquet in Paris discovered another opium derivative—codeine. Later in the 19th century, heroin was first prepared in Germany. The latter is the most effective analgesic of all the opiate derivatives and also has caused the most human suffering through misuse.

It was during the 19th century, when opiate derivatives were being discovered, that the hypodermic syringe was developed. This technical innovation resulted in increased use of morphine and later heroin—with an attendant rise in drug dependency.

The language of medicine often helps us follow the trail of medical thought and practice. Here are the etymologic origins of opium and its derivatives: The word *opium* is from the Greek *opion*, which refers to the juice of the poppy. Camphorated tincture of opium is called *paregoric*, from a Greek term denoting "consoling and soothing," certainly an appropriate appellation for a medication that can staunch dysentery (Haubrich, p. 161). *Laudanum* comes from a Latin word describing a Cyprian shrub (Partridge, p. 340), although Weekley (p. 827) suggests that Paracelsus may have used the word to describe his opium-laced elixir because the word *laud* means "praise" in Latin.

From the Greek god of dreams, Morpheus, comes the word *morphine*, referring to its hypnotic properties. Next came *codeine*, from the Greek word *kodeia*, meaning "head," referring to the "head" of the opium poppy. I find the most ironic etymology of all to be that of the word *heroin*, which comes from Heroin, a trademark registered in 1898 by Friedrich Bayer & Co. The origin is the Greek word *heros*, meaning "hero," connoting the "high" that can make the user feel superhuman.

In my professional life, I have encountered all of the opiate variants described above. Paregoric, camphorated tincture of opium, is a seldom used remedy for recalcitrant diarrhea; in the early years of my practice, I prescribed this drug from time to time and was impressed with its effectiveness. I carried a morphine vial in my black house-call bag and found it to be literally lifesaving a few times when faced with a pulmonary edema patient at home and far from the hospital. Codeine is today one of our most effective antitussives. In World War II, it was used extensively by U.S. soldiers (presumably because of some mysterious endemic idiopathic cough), who referred to it as "GI gin." More recently, working in a clinic caring for many homeless persons, I have seen the devastation caused by heroin in its various forms of administration.

To return to our story, in the United States the 1914 Harrison Act criminalized drug addiction. Opiates were available only by prescription, thus greatly increasing the monetary value of illicit drugs. Supplying a narcotic drug to an addicted person became illegal, resulting in the arraignment of approximately 25,000 American physicians and subsequent imprisonment of 3,000 of them (Porter, p. 665).

Since 1914, America has engaged in its "war on drugs" with astonishingly little success. From time to time, a physician is arrested for "illegal prescribing of narcotics," but such instances are uncommon, and most medical narcotic use is for "laudable" purposes. The narcotic problem long ago moved from the doctor's office to the streets, airports, cargo ships, and impoverished countries where the opium poppy is an economically vital cash crop.

Ergot

Many family physicians have special areas of interest, such as sports medicine, adolescent health care, or geriatrics. My specialty has been headaches, and at one time headache patients constituted almost a third of my practice. Hence, in the days before the "triptans," I prescribed ergot preparations for hundreds of patients, and I still consider them to be useful—and under-used—medications. In addition to their clinical utility, the ergot derivatives have a very colorful history, as well as being part of a confusing etymologic controversy.

Ergot arises naturally from a fungus, *Claviceps purpura*, which grows on grasses and cereal grains, notably rye. A 600 BCE Assyrian tablet describes the fungus as a "noxious pustule in the ear of grain." The agent is a vasoconstrictor with oxytocic properties that have been recognized since very early times. *Ergot* is an Old French word meaning "cock's spur," alluding to the shape of the fungus as it grows on the grain.

Ergotism is caused by a chronic overdose of ergot, and the manifestations chiefly reflect peripheral vasoconstriction. An early symptom is a burning sensation in the hands and feet, after which the most peripheral tissues become dry and black because of impaired circulation. In extreme cases, fingers and toes become mummified and fall off. In addition, pregnant women can suffer abortions.

Ackerknecht records that Galen was familiar with the disease but that ergotism was not found in the inhabitants of ancient Greece or Rome as rye was not part of their diet (p. 139). In the Middle Ages, however, ergotism was a significant problem, notably in northern Europe. Ergotism tends to come during damp periods (a common climactic condition during medieval times) when the fungus grows luxuriantly on grain. The disease is also prevalent in times of food shortage, when grain becomes the chief food consumed. The combination of these factors—damp weather and famine—contributed to the epidemic of ergotism in the Middle Ages. In that era, the burning sensation of ergotism came to be called St. Anthony's fire. Why?

St. Anthony of Padua (1195–1231) was a Portuguese Franciscan who, in a vision, received the infant Jesus in his arms. He was canonized in the year after his death and today is especially invoked for the recovery of things lost. He is also patron saint of amputees, animals, boatmen, domestic animals, expectant mothers, fishermen, harvests, horses, mariners, oppressed people, paupers, sailors, scholars, swineherds, travel hostesses, and travelers. St. Anthony's relics are preserved at the basilica in Padua, Italy.

Somehow, ergot sufferers discovered that their burning and other symptoms abated if they made a pilgrimage to St. Anthony's Basilica in Italy. The reason? As they made the sojourn, they reduced their consumption of contaminated rye products and ate the greater variety of foods available in sunny Italy (Goodman and Gilman, p. 872). As their daily consumption of tainted grains ceased, the manifestations of ergotism miraculously improved.

The Middle Ages probably was not the last time the world saw ergotism. Matossian makes a plausible case that the hysteria of the 1692 Salem witch trials might have been the result of ergotism (1). She notes that the symptoms of the young "witches" seem to match some of the manifestations of ergotism: feelings of burning or being pinched, visual hallucinations, and out-of-body sensations. All of these could have been caused by arterial vasospasm. One report at the time describes red sacramental bread; bread with a high ergot content tends to be cherry red in color. We will never know with certainty whether ergot caused the 1692 witchcraft phenomena, but reflection on the event is a stimulating exercise in retrospective diagnosis, which I will discuss further in chapter 9.

Matossian postulates that the beginning of the French Revolution in 1789 might also be attributed to ergot poisoning. Trouble began as panicked peasants fled to the forests and armed themselves with pitchforks and clubs. Three weeks of riots marked the beginning of the revolt that brought down the monarchy. Matossian has discovered that the weather in the spring and early summer of 1789 was wet and cold—the very conditions most favorable to the growth of rye fungus. Furthermore, shortly before the uprising, the peasants had begun to eat flour ground from the summer's rye crop. To make matters worse, there were rumors that the aristocrats were sending bandits to confiscate the rye crop, which would have caused starvation among the peasants. Matossian concludes, "These people weren't rebelling. They were terrified" (2).

What about the etymological confusion? First of all, there is more than one St. Anthony. In Egypt, St. Anthony of the Desert, aka St. Anthony the Great (251–356), predated St. Anthony of Padua by nine centuries. St. Anthony the Great gave all his worldly possessions to the poor and spent the rest of his life in monastic prayer in the desert. Then, in 1090, the father of a young man with ergotism vowed on the tomb of St. Anthony of the Desert that he would henceforth devote his resources to the aid of ergotism victims if only his son would be cured. St. Anthony of the Desert then became the patron saint of ergotism sufferers. Also, during the Middle Ages, there were a number of epidemics called *ignis sacer* (holy fire) or St. Anthony's fire—names that are not illogical given the hyper-religiosity of the times. Some, but not all, of these epidemics were ergotism; other causes included erysipelas, scurvy, and anthrax (Ackerknecht, p. 139).

Today, you may find articles or dictionaries that define St. Anthony's fire as ergotism, erysipelas, or both. For the record, I looked up St. Anthony's fire in my *Stedman's Electronic Medical Dictionary*. The entry states, without equivocation, that St. Anthony's fire is a synonym for ergotism, and the historical origin listed is the Egyptian monk St. Anthony of the Desert.

And what about ergotism today? The chief use of ergot is in headache therapy. The disease ergotism, rare in the 21st century, is most likely to be seen in patients who overuse ergotamine-containing medications for migraine headache, as reported by Zavaleta et al. (3).

Quinine

In chapter 2, I discussed malaria—a disease that afflicted much of the ancient world, notably in areas where mosquito vectors were prevalent. Early practitioners often applied the popular remedies for fever—bleeding and purging—measures that were less than helpful for persons with malaria-induced anemia (Cartwright, p. 143). Then, sometime in the early 17th century, the Spanish conquerors in Peru learned that the Andean natives had recognized the therapeutic properties of the bark of the "fever tree," now called *Cinchona calisaya*. In the native language, Quechua, the word for the bark of the tree was *quina* or *quina-quina*, meaning "bark of bark." Cartwright (p. 143) describes what may be an etymologic misadventure. Some thought that the bark, cinchona, came from the name of the wife of the Spanish Governor of Peru, the Countess of Chinchon. Legend holds that in 1742 she used the native remedy to overcome a febrile illness and subsequently shipped a supply of the bark to Spain. We now know that the name of the tree and the medicine came from the Native American language and that by 1742 the bark had been used in Europe for at least 100 years.

By 1820, the active principle, now named quinine, had been extracted from the "Peruvian bark." In 1833, quinidine, an alkaloid of cinchona, was discovered and was so named because as an isomer, it is a sort of "quin*oi-dine*" (Haubrich, p. 187). By 1850, quinine was widely used for malaria prophylaxis.

Quinine became especially significant in World War II, when many Allied troops were sent to malaria-infested areas. Under the pressure of the war effort, Edwin H. Land (do you recall the Polaroid Land Camera?) led a research team that discovered a way to make quinine without the use of Peruvian bark.

What is quinine? Bateman and Dyson describe quinine as a "general protoplasmic poison" that is toxic to many microorganisms, including the malarial plasmodia (4). The drug can cause headache, vasodilation, sweating, gastrointestinal disturbances, tinnitus, visual and auditory symptoms, and thrombocytopenia. But today, since few of us will prescribe quinine for malaria prophylaxis or therapy, what is the significance of the drug's toxic properties?

First of all, the drug is rumored to be an abortifacient; self-poisoning can follow the consumption of large quantities taken in an effort to terminate a pregnancy. Also, quinine is occasionally used to "cut" heroin for illicit use, resulting in inadvertent toxicity in users. What's more, quinine is often prescribed to treat nocturnal leg cramps, a benefit attributed to the drug's property of prolonging the refractory period of skeletal muscle.

A more quaint use is the addition of quinine to seltzer water to produce tonic water, a custom that probably began with the British Raj in India, who mixed quinine tonic water with gin for its healthful effects. This continues today with tonic water and bitter lemon beverages. However, such use is not without risk. Brasic reports a case of quinine-induced thrombocytopenia precipitated by "voluminous consumption" of tonic water to relieve nocturnal leg cramps (5).

Barbiturates

In 1863, two chemists at the Friedrich Bayer Company in Germany (which would later give the world aspirin) isolated a chemical that turned out to have hypnotic, sedative, and anticonvulsive actions. The name may come from the German *Barbitursäuer*, from St. Barbara's Day, when the compound was discovered. St. Barbara is the patron saint of artillery officers, and the tavern where the Bayer team toasted their new discovery was a favorite of artillery officers. Fortuine (p. 258) adds an intriguing footnote to the tale: "A company representative has stated that the name derived from a Munich café waitress named Barbara, who had often donated urine specimens for the investigation." Another legend is that "Barbara" was the girlfriend of one of the chemists.

For those who relish etymologic controversy, Pepper (p. 100) has another theory. He holds that the "barba" part of barbiturate comes from Latin *barba*, meaning "beard," and *-urate* refers to uric acid. Pepper does not mention girlfriends or saints, and I personally prefer the more colorful explanations.

The first compound discovered was barbital, introduced in 1903 as Veronal—the trade name referring to Verona, Italy, where Juliet swallowed a sleep potion. (Romeo did so also, but unlike Juliet, he failed to awaken from the drug-induced state.)

Then came phenobarbital, marketed as Luminal, from the Latin word *lumen*, meaning "light." I have never been too sure how a sedative hypnotic drug brings one to light; it seems that the opposite might occur. However, I do recall that in the early 1960s we treated hypertension with 15-mg phenobarbital tablets taken three times daily.

Then came pentobarbital (Nembutal), an excellent hypnotic widely used a generation or two ago. This was followed by amobarbital (Amytal), and eventually some 2,500 barbiturate compounds were synthesized, of which some 50 were eventually brought to market.

Today, in the state of Oregon, assisted suicide is legal. The patient who chooses this option will (after satisfying the many strict legal requirements) eventually be given a prescription for barbiturates.

Aspirin

Inexpensive, potent, and possessing a reasonable spectrum of side effects, aspirin is one of the world's most cost-effective medications. We use the drug to relieve many types of pain, to combat the inflammation of arthritis, and to treat acute heart attacks. It is a seemingly "magic" treatment for osteoid osteoma and in low doses can help prevent stroke recurrence. Aspirin represents a classic story of a folk remedy that has become a widely used modern drug.

Aspirin's precursors have been used for more than two millennia. Before salicylic compounds were discovered in the bark and leaves of plants, Hippocrates (460–377 BCE) treated fever and labor pain with willow extract, the ancient Egyptians recognized the analgesic properties of myrtle leaves, and Native Americans chewed willow bark as a folk remedy for various ailments. In 18th century England, it was believed that willow helped reduce fever because both fever and willow are found in damp areas.

In the 1820s and 1830s, salicylic acid was derived by adding an acid to an extract of the *Salicaceae* family of willows and poplar. Later, a naturally occurring salicylic acid (no added acid needed) was discovered in a species of the *Spiraea* genus, meadowsweet. In 1853, acetylsalicylic acid was formed by adding an acetyl group to the salicylic acid. Then, in 1897, Felix Hoffmann, an industrial chemist employed by the Friedrich Bayer Company, found a practical way of making a stable, solid form of acetylsalicylic acid which could be produced as tablets. Hoffmann's father, who suffered from severe arthritis, was treated with the new drug, reporting superior pain relief and fewer side effects.

In 1899, Bayer set out to promote their new discovery, which became the world's first medicine to be sold in tablet form and eventually the world's largest-selling over-the-counter medication (Gershen, p. 119). First, a name was needed. Bayer chose the word *aspirin*: *a-* to denote the addition of the acetyl group, *spririn* to indicate the *Spiraea* genus, and *-in* as a commonly used suffix for medications.

Because acetylsalicylic acid is a chemical that can be readily manufactured by any pharmaceutical company, the name of the drug was quite important. Bayer received a trademark on the word *aspirin* in 1889. Following World War I, and probably somewhat as a result of the ill feelings engendered, Bayer lost trademark protection in the U.S., Great Britain, and France. As a result of a U.S. Supreme Court decision in 1919, the word *aspirin* became a generic term in the English language, a fate that today certainly concerns the makers of Kleenex tissues, Xerox copiers, and Scotch Tape. Today, Aspirin is a registered trademark of Bayer AG in Germany and more than 80 other countries, but not in the U.S.

Penicillin

In chapter 1, I discussed the discovery of penicillin as a milestone in medical history, and a grand event it was. Penicillin was the first of the bacteriocidal antibiotics and, in a sense, is the gold standard against which we measure all that have been discovered since. But penicillin languished for more than a decade between its discovery as a laboratory curiosity and its use as a life-saving antimicrobial. This is the story.

We all know that in 1928, British bacteriologist Alexander Fleming, described by Weiss (p. 76) as "not the neatest of laboratory workers," returned from vacation and began to clean up a pile of plates that he had cultured before his departure. The historic plate, showing a mold contaminant that had caused lysis in nearby bacteria, had been thrown into a tray of disinfectant. "That's funny," said Fleming, referring to the mold-bacteria phenomenon, and he retrieved the plate, which fortunately had not been submerged in disinfectant. This set in motion a chain of events in which Fleming, along with others described below, received a Nobel Prize, making him one of the very few Nobel laureates in medicine whose name is known outside the walls of academia.

It seems that Dr. Fleming may have had the ability to recognize the significance of a chance observation, but he lacked what was needed to exploit his finding. He published the results of his studies in the *British Journal of Experimental Pathology*, he presented his findings at scientific meetings, and he tried unsuccessfully to persuade physicians to use penicillin. Lax tells of Fleming's unconvincing presentation skills, inadequate experimental design, inconclusive experimental results, and "miserly" literary style (6).

In 1939, Howard Florey, professor of pathology at Oxford University, and his colleague Earnest Chain resumed work on penicillin. In 1940, a classically designed study looked at what happened to mice infected with large doses of streptococci. Half were injected with penicillin and lived; the other half received no therapy and died.

Shortly after the mouse experiment, World War II began and the development of penicillin took on great urgency. Penicillin was grown in broth in bedpans and subsequently in specially designed ceramic culture trays. The few units of penicillin developed were precious and were sometimes retrieved from the urine of patients who had been given the drug. One such patient was a local policeman, and Goodman and Gilman report that, "It is said that an Oxford professor referred to penicillin as a remarkable substance, grown in bedpans and purified by passage through the Oxford Police Force" (p. 1130).

As France fell to the German invasion, Florey and his colleagues feared that Britain might be invaded. If so, they planned to destroy their work rather than have it fall into Nazi hands. As a precaution, they smeared their jackets with *Penicillium* spore so that their discovery could travel with them if they were forced to flee (6).

The U.S. entered the war in 1941. Florey and colleague Norman Heatley flew to the U.S. to meet with American scientists, who had begun work on penicillin as a high priority. The epicenter of work was the Northern Regional Research Laboratories of the Department of Agriculture in Peoria, Illinois. One interesting sidelight is the story of "Moldy Mary" Hunt, an assistant assigned to find molded fruit to test for strains of *Penicillium*. Hunt found the most luxuriantly productive strain of mold growing on a cantaloupe in a Peoria fruit market.

In World War II, penicillin saved the lives of countless Allied troops. Production capabilities increased rapidly, and from an early meager output, the U.S. production of penicillin reached 222 trillion units (148 tons) in 1950.

Fleming, Florey, and Chain shared the 1945 Nobel Prize for Physiology or Medicine. At Fleming's death, flower vendors in Barcelona decorated the tablet erected when Fleming had visited their city, and on Greek islands, flags flew at half-staff. These were all quite generous tributes to a man who delayed and almost "disinfected" one of the epic discoveries of the 20th century.

Short Tales About Selected Remedies

Vitamins

Vitamins are naturally occurring substances and are not really remedies, unless one happens to have a vitamin deficiency. I have included vitamins here because I find their story interesting. In the early years of the 20th century, observers became aware that persons eating a diet composed chiefly of white (polished) rice were much more likely to develop beriberi than those who ate "rough" unpolished rice. Something seemed to be missing in the white rice. In a 1905 experiment that would hardly be approved today, William Fletcher (1874–1938) studied two groups of inmates in a Kuala Lumpur prison, feeding one group a diet high in polished rice while the other group ate "rough" rice. The prisoners eating polished rice had a much higher incidence of beriberi than those eating unpolished rice (Porter, p. 554).

The results from Malaysia and separate observations of beriberi among Norwegian sailors on long voyages were followed by animal experiments, eventually showing that quite small quantities of "accessory food factors" could prevent beriberi, as well as rickets, scurvy, and pellagra.

The first vitamin isolated was discovered in 1911 by a Polish biochemist with the euphonious name Casimir Funk (1884–1967). Funk's discovery was an amine of nicotinic acid, which could prevent beriberi. He coined the word "vitamine," indicating that he considered the amine to be vital to life.

In 1913, a substance called vitamin A was discovered. Credit goes to Elmer McCollum (1879–1967) and his team at the University of Wisconsin (Sebastian, p. 751). As subsequent vitamins were discovered, they were assigned the letters B (eight of which are numbered), C, D, and so forth. The alphabetical aberration was vitamin K, named in 1935 by Danish biochemist Henrick Dam (1895–1976). Vitamin K helps prevent a hemorrhagic disorder and hence is the *koagulation* vitamin (Haubrich, p. 245). There are also vitamin wannabes—such as U and O.

Along the way, specifically in 1920, the terminal *e* was dropped from vitamine when it was found that not all vitamins were amines. Today, we in the developed world consume huge quantities of vitamins, while controversy rages as to whether this one or that is really useful in preventing heart disease, cancer, or various manifestations of aging. Strangely, it all began with camel dung, as I describe next.

Amines

The story of the amine group (NH_2), the basis of the gas ammonia (NH_3), begins in North Africa about the fourth century BCE, the time of Alexander the Great. At the shrine of Jupiter Ammon, near the Libyan city of Ammonia, visitors inside the temple warmed themselves around fires made with the customary fuel—dried camel dung (Shipley, p. 1945). And why not? Firewood was unavailable in the desert. American pioneers in the 1800s used "chips" of cattle and buffalo, and today in many desert villages, animal dung is dried for use as fuel.

Back to the story. Inside the temple, the years' accumulation of smoke caused a powder to form in the ceiling. This was called *sal ammoniac*, or the salt of Ammon (Gershen, p. 2001). Fast forward to 1774, when Joseph Priestley, Unitarian minister and chemist who later discovered oxygen, found that adding an acid to *sal ammoniac* yielded a pungent gas. With this discovery, science was on its way to understanding one of the important building blocks of all proteins—the amines—and to Funk's discovery of his "vitamine."

Nitrogen Mustard

On April 22, 1915, chemical warfare using toxic gas was formally introduced into the world. The place was the city of Ypres, a small Flemish market town just over the border from France. The setting was the Western Front of World War I, and the event was the release of chlorine gas by German troops. As the gas wafted over the Allied lines, there were more than 5,000 casualties (Weiss, p. 125).

Later came subsequent generations of poison gas—phosgene and eventually mustard gas. Mustard gas, however, did not merely poison the lungs of those who inhaled it. Some exposed soldiers developed bone marrow aplasia. The poison gas seemed to attack cells that produced blood cells.

If nitrogen mustard can attack blood cells in healthy persons, might it also do so—beneficially—in persons with too many cells, such as patients with lymphoma? In 1942, nitrogen mustard was first used to treat a patient with lymphoma. We now know that nitrogen mustard is an alkylating agent that modifies cellular DNA. Since the 1940s, we have discovered better and safer alkylating agents—chlorambucil, melphalan, and busulphan—as well as other classes of chemotherapeutic drugs. But the first suggestion that a drug could reduce harmful cell production can be traced to a Flemish battlefield enveloped by a cloud of toxic gas.

Isoniazid

Isoniazid has been a mainstay in the treatment of tuberculosis. It is still quite a useful drug, having three of my favorite characteristics: It is old, cheap, and relatively safe. To make a long story short, in 1952 two companies—Squibb and Hoffmann-La Roche—independently and coincidentally announced the discovery of a new antituberculous drug, isonicotinic acid hydrazide.

In a moment of wisdom that avoided years of agony and millions of dollars in litigation, the two companies agreed upon a novel approach to resolve the conflict. They decided to drop the dated notes of their investigators into a hat. They agreed that the patent rights would go to the company with the earlier date and that the other company would have a royalty-free right to manufacture and sell isoniazid. In the drawing, Hoffman-La Roche was the winner—by a few days in the dated notes.

But wisdom is not always rewarded. When the patent application was filed, there was a third claim that predated even those of the two major companies. Only a "use" patent was granted, and neither company received major profits from the venture.

There was one bright note, however. In 1955, the Albert Lasker Medical Research Award was presented to both Squibb and Hoffmann-La Roche, the first pharmaceutical companies ever to be so honored (Bordley, p. 461).

A Potpourri of Drug Names

As we close this chapter, here is a short list of intriguing drug names:

In 1942, Ayerst needed a brand name for its new product containing estrogenic hormones. The source of the compound was the urine of pregnant mares. Hence, a logical name for the new medications was Premarin (Fortuine, p. 317).

In 1943, a young girl sustained an open fracture of the leg, which became infected. Cultures of the infection yielded a substance with, ironically, antimicrobial properties. The cultured organism was named *Bacillus subtilis*. The young girl was named Margaret Tracy. The antibiotic produced from the culture material was named bacitracin, in honor of Margaret.

Also in the 1940s, chemists at the University of Wisconsin were working on a problem. It seemed that cattle eating moldy silage made from sweet clover suffered severe bleeding problems and sometimes died of internal hemorrhage. Studies showed that the active agent was a coumarin derivative. The first patented coumarin product was dicoumarol, patented in 1941. But subsequent efforts yielded a superior drug, released as warfarin (Coumadin) in 1948. Why was the drug named *warfarin*? WARF stands for Wisconsin Alumni Research Foundation, and -*arin* denotes its relationship to coumarin.

In 1950, nystatin was developed to treat *Candida* infections. The drug is derived from bacteria found in the garden of a friend of one of the researchers; the friend's name was Nourse, and so the organism was termed *Streptomyces noursei*. The drug itself, nystatin, was named to commemorate its place of origin: the New York State Public Health Department.

References

1. Matossian MK. The crucible of Salem: witchcraft, ergo ergotism. *MD Magazine.* November 1992:85–93.
2. Matossian MK. Ergot and the French Revolution: Chapter 6: The Great Fear of 1789. In: *Poisons of the Past: Molds, Epidemics and History.* Matossian MK, ed. New Haven, CT: Yale University Press; 1989.
3. Zavaleta EG, Fernandez BB, Grove MK, Kaye MD. St. Anthony's fire (ergotamine induced leg ischemia)—a case report and review of the literature. *Angiology.* 2001;52:349–356.
4. Bateman DN, Dyson EH. Quinine toxicity. *Adverse Drug React Acute Poisoning Rev.* 1986;5:215–233.

5. Brasic JR. Quinine-induced thrombocytopenia in a 64-year-old man who consumed tonic water to relieve nocturnal leg cramps. *Mayo Clin Proc.* 2001;76;863–866.
6. Lax E. *The Mold in Dr. Florey's Coat: The Story of the Penicillin Miracle.* New York, NY: Henry Holt; 2004.

Part Two
The Heritage and Culture of Medicine

4
Medical Words and Phrases

Words dwell in our minds like insects in a forest, or, indeed, like the countless friendly organisms that inhabit the human body. We could scarcely exist without them. They illustrate what one might call cultural Darwinism. New words arrive—borne by conquest, commerce, or science—and supplant their predecessors. But the old words never fade entirely away. They linger faintly in the shadows, understudies hoping to be called back on stage.

John Train (1)

Some people collect coins or postage stamps. Others collect Depression-era glass dishes or old guns. I collect words. My bookshelves at home groan from the weight of word origin books, and I advise young medical students to look up the source of each new word they encounter. My fascination with words began with the encouragement of my high school Latin teacher, Miss Irwin, and continued into college, where I began to keep notebooks of new words and—just as important—their origins. When I entered medical school, I was delighted to find a whole new world of medical terms, most of sufficiently recent coinage that the origin of a term could be traced. For me, some medical terms have remarkably absorbing histories. This chapter tells some of those tales.

About Medical Words

Where do medical words come from? The origin of most from old Greek and Latin is a fortuitous, if not intentional, circumstance because both these tongues are "completed" languages, not subject to capricious additions, subtractions, or modifications of words. Some scientific names, notably microbiologic terms, were created to honor individuals who made important contributions to science. Consider *Coxiella burnetii* (the cause of Q fever), named for scientists Herald R. Cox and Sir Frank Macfarlane Burnet, who identified the organism in 1937. Other medical words and phrases have been appropriated from a variety of sources, such as mythology (e.g., *hermaphroditism*), other languages (e.g., *mittelschmerz*), or literature (Alice in Wonderland syndrome). And a few of the terms we use today are simply everyday English words such as *belly* and *gut*.

The influence of ancient Greek and Latin on medical terms is profound. The historical reason that both are used relates to events about two millennia ago and earlier. The early Greeks evolved a language that included many words that came from lands they conquered. Maleska (p. 86) points out that when the Greeks conquered Persia, part of their booty was words of Aryan or Indo-Iranian origin. Eventually, the Roman Empire conquered Greece and brought home the jewels of Hellenic culture and scholarship, including their language. The Romans also brought back Greek physicians, whose clinical skills were much superior to those of Roman practitioners. Romans of the patrician class adopted Greek as an elitist second language, helping to meld elements of both languages.

In what must have been an astoundingly tedious exercise, Butler examined the sources of medical words in the 24th edition of *Dorland's Illustrated Medical Dictionary* (2). The distribution of origins is as follows: Greek alone, 58.5%; Latin alone, 21.7%; English, 2.9%; proper names, 1.5%; French, 1.1%; Arabic, 0.6%; German, 0.46%; Spanish, 0.27%; and Italian, 0.11%. The remainder are hybrids or are from various other sources.

I offer this personal comment on the German contribution to medical terminology and science. In the late 19th and early 20th century, some aspiring physicians earnestly studied German as a means of reading the most modern scientific papers, which were likely to come from Germany—such as the report of the new x-rays discovered in 1895 by *Herr* Roentgen and the "magic bullet" discovery of Paul Ehrlich in 1907. In 1954, I paid my dues at the time by taking a college course in scientific German. Today, all important scientific papers are sooner or later published in English, and (probably owing to the inherent complexity of Teutonic word structure) few German words have survived into modern scientific use.

To get us started at looking at medical words, let us examine five everyday clinical terms: *medicine, patient, doctor, physician*, and *professional*. I cover these first in this chapter because we should all know these terms intimately and use them correctly.

Medicine comes directly from the Latin *medicia*, and in Roman days *medicus* meant "healer." Martí-Ibáñez (p. 6) explains that the root *med* means "to think," or meditate, and hence medicine connotes both healing and thinking.

Patient has nothing at all to do with "patiently" waiting to see the doctor. The word comes from the Latin *patientia*, which comes from the verb *pati*, meaning "to suffer." Use of the word to describe someone who seeks medical care can be traced to Middle English.

The Latin word *docere*, meaning "to teach," is the source of the word *doctor*. Hence, a doctor is a teacher who may hold a degree in medicine, religion, law, or other learned discipline. The word *docent*, describing (for example) a person who leads educational tours in museums, comes from the same Latin root.

According to Pepper (p. 119), *physician* comes from the ancient Latin word *physicus*, meaning "one who studied physical philosophy," "for in the field of physical philosophy, medicine was the zenith." The word came into English in the 14th century as a variant of the French word *physicien* to describe a practitioner of the healing arts.

Lastly, the physician is a *professional*, the word coming from Latin through Old French to indicate "one who makes vows or a public declaration," as one would when being received into a religious order. Physicians take as their public declaration the Oath of Hippocrates (see chapter 1) or the Oath of Geneva. Sometime in the 16th century, the meaning of the word was broadened to mean an occupation in which one "professes" to be skillful, such as professional plumber or basketball player. There is also the current connotation that a professional—such as a professional athlete—is not an amateur. The physician is a professional and probably a doctor, but never a provider. *Provider*, from the Latin *providere*, means "one who prepares or supplies." Physicians are healers and teachers but must resist being designated *provisioners* or, even worse, *PCPs* (i.e., primary care providers) (3).

Origins

Although most medical words come from other earlier languages, saying this is so is not quite enough. The words we use today found their way into common clinical use and onto the pages of medical dictionaries by varied pathways. Here are some of them.

Mythology

As we begin to look at word origins, mythology seems a good place to start because many myths predate recorded history and are the quintessential "stories around the campfire."

We all know the Achilles' tendon, which attaches to the heel bone (*os calcis*). In myths surrounding the Trojan War, the infant Achilles was dipped in the river Styx by his mother, Thetis, making him invulnerable to injury wherever the waters touched him. But as he was dipped, his mother held him by the heel, which remained dry and hence vulnerable. Later, Achilles was killed when an arrow fired by Paris struck him in his unprotected heel.

In the 16th century, Vesalius named the first cervical vertebra the atlas, because it supports the skull. The choice was metaphorically appropriate because in the ancient Greek myth, Atlas, one of the Titans, took part in the War of the Titans and was subsequently condemned by Zeus to hold the world on his shoulders. His home was named the Atlas Mountains in Africa, consistent with the myth that Atlas supported the heavens (Evans IH, p. 57). Well and good, but why do we call a collection of maps an atlas? Also in the 16th century, French cartographer Gerardus Mercator (1512–1594) published a collection of maps with a cover depicting Atlas holding up the world. Since then, a book of maps has been called an atlas (Hendrickson, p. 245).

One of the 12 Olympic gods, Aphrodite (called Venus by the Romans and Ishtar by the Mesopotamians) was renowned for her beauty, charm, and, to be frank, her sexuality. She was a seductress who occasionally used potions to help charm her paramours, giving us the word *aphrodisiac*. From her Roman counterpart, Venus, we get the word *venereal*.

Aphrodite had a child named Eros (called Cupid by the Romans), the god of love, who was the source of the word *erotic*. Her second child was Hymen, the god of marriage, whose medical cognate describes a slip of tissue at the vaginal orifice, with profound significance in matrimonial matters in some cultures.

Aphrodite had a son by Hermes, the Olympic god of commerce, shepherds, and poets. Named for both his parents, Hermaphroditus grew to be a handsome lad, so attractive that the nymph Salmacis fell in love with him and prayed that her spirit and body might be merged with his as one. Her prayers were answered, and since then any person who has both male and female sexual characteristics is called a *hermaphrodite*.

Yet another son of the very popular and fertile Aphrodite was Priapus, whose father was Dionysus. The god of fertility and reproductive potency, Priapus served as the protector of farmers and shepherds, whose livelihood often depends on the fecundity of their livestock. That Priapus was the god of procreation has been made quite obvious in many statues, and his name has been given to the medical syndrome of *priapism*.

Pan was the Greek god of the wild animals and forests, a playful and libidinous imp with the horns, tail, and feet of a goat. He was a mischievous goblin who liked to leap from behind trees to terrify persons walking in the woods. From these pranks comes the word *panic*, describing a terrifying sense of anxiety.

Proteus was a Greek sea god who could change his shape at will. Today, we have the Proteus syndrome, a rare disorder with hamartomatous manifestations in multiple body systems, not unlike neurofibromatosis. Joseph Merrick, better known as "The Elephant Man," is now believed by some to have had the Proteus syndrome.

The word *sphincter* comes from the mythological Sphinx, a monstrous being with the head of a woman and the body of a lion. The Sphinx guarded the entry to the city of Thebes and asked each person who entered to solve a riddle: What moves on four legs in the morning, two at noon, and three in the evening? Those who failed to solve the riddle were promptly strangled to death. In the end, the riddle was solved by Oedipus: The answer is man, who crawls as an infant, walks upright when an adult, and uses a cane in old age. The Sphinx, enraged that someone had solved the riddle, destroyed itself. All this strangling is why we now call a circular muscle that can squeeze tightly a *sphincter*.

Some Word Roots That Helped Me Survive Anatomy

Perhaps nowhere in the study of medicine is etymology as helpful as in the study of anatomy. Today, gross anatomy is considered a "completed discipline," with nothing new to discover, but since the time of Vesalius anatomists have named many body organs by likening them to items that seemed to have similar shapes or functions. Here is a list of some of them:

Anatomical Term	Word Origin
Acetabulum	Vinegar cup (Latin)
Biceps	Two heads (Latin); also triceps, quadriceps
Cervix	Neck (Latin)
Clavicle	Key (Latin); named for the shape of the bone
Colon	Hollow (Greek)
Cortex	Bark (Latin)
Deltoid	Delta (Greek): the Greek letter is shaped like a triangle.
Disc	Flat dish (Greek)
Falx	Sickle (Latin)
Follicle	Small sac (Latin)
Fossa	Trench (Latin)
Glans	Acorn (Latin)
Incus	Anvil (Latin)
Infundibulum	Funnel (Latin)
Malleus	Hammer (Latin)
Patella	Dish (Latin)
Pelvis	Basin (Latin)
Penis	Tail (Latin); not anatomically precise, but memorable
Phalanx	Line of soldiers (Greek)
Placenta	Cake (Latin)
Pons	Bridge (Latin)
Rectum	Straight (Latin)
Sella	Saddle (Latin)
Stapes	Stirrup (Latin)
Tibia	Flute (Latin), from the shape of the bone
Uvula	Little grape (Latin)
Vagina	Sheath (Latin)
Vas	Vessel (Latin)
Xiphoid	Sword (Greek)

Places in the Medical Dictionary

A surprisingly large number of medical terms contain geographic names, usually denoting where a disease was first found or where something noteworthy happened.

Medical Term	Significance
Bornholm disease	Bornholm is a small Danish island in the Baltic Sea and the home of patients from whom scientists first recovered the virus that causes epidemic pleurodynia.
Coxsackie viruses	These are a group of enteroviruses first isolated from a patient who lived in Coxsackie, a small town in the Hudson Valley in upstate New York.
Dum Dum fever	This synonym for visceral leishmaniasis (aka *kala-azar*) comes from the town in India where William Leishman discovered the parasite in 1903 (Fortuine, p. 262).
Epsom Salts	This commercial name for magnesium sulphate, a laxative, was first found by evaporation of bitter-tasting water from a mineral spring at Epsom in Surrey, England. Evans IH (p. 380) explains that the properties of the water were discovered in 1618 when a farmer discovered that, even in times of drought, his cows refused to drink from the spring.
Hanta virus	The source of this name is a river in Korea.
Norwalk virus	The stool specimen that first yielded the virus came from persons at a school in Norwalk, Ohio. Norwalk virus is a member of the genus *Norovirus* of the family *Caliciviridae*.
Milk of Magnesia	Milk of Magnesia, the commercial name for the laxative agent magnesium hydroxide, comes from the town of Magnesia, in northwestern Turkey. In 1831, a French chemist isolated magnesium in ore found in the area.
Miltown	This proprietary name for the tranquilizer meprobamate comes from a village, Milltown, located near the home of Wallace Laboratories in New Brunswick, New Jersey. Wallace Laboratories used the town name as a code name for the drug while it was being developed prior to its release in 1955. The company then kept the word *Miltown*, with only a slight change in spelling, as a brand name (Fortuine, p. 263).

Medical Term	Significance
Minamata disease	In the 1950s, Minamata Bay in Japan became polluted with mercury. Inhabitants of the area, whose dietary staple was locally caught seafood, sustained dementia and neurologic damage owing to chronic methyl mercury poisoning.
Plaster of Paris	The gypsum from which Plaster of Paris was made was quarried in Montmartre, a Paris neighborhood that is now a favorite of tourists (Pepper, p. 148).
Rocky Mountain Spotted Fever	This tickborne rickettsial disease was first discovered in 1896 in Idaho, where the rash was called "black measles." Today, the disease is more likely to be found in persons living in North Carolina than in Idaho.
Tularemia	Tularemia, which has some similarities to plague, was named in 1919 by epidemiologist Edward Francis (1872–1957). The name commemorates Tulare County in central California, where the disease was first identified (Haubrich, p. 234). Tulare County is named for tule, a reed growing wild in marshy areas. Tule grows so abundantly in that area of California that the phrase "out in the tulies" is a synonym for "rural."

Words From Other Languages

Almost all our medical words, of course, come from languages other than English. In this section, I will present a few words that entered our clinical vocabulary which do not have ancient Greek or Latin roots. As indicated in the tabulation of word origins above, the number is not large. Here are some examples:

Beriberi is a classical disease name coming from another language. The word comes from the Singhalese word meaning "I cannot" or "weak," and the repetition is used for emphasis, indicating extreme weakness. Such repetition for emphasis is common in Asian languages (Haubrich, p. 29). As described in chapter 3, the disease is a polyneuropathy found in persons whose dietary staple is polished rice with a resultant niacin deficiency.

Bezoar comes from a Persian word *padzahr*, meaning "antidote." A bezoar is a concretion—classically, a ball of hair—sometimes found in the stomach or intestines of animals or humans. Most prized by the ancient Persians was the *padzahr* from the wild mountain goat, which was believed to have therapeutic properties as a universal antidote.

Dengue may be a contraction of "dandy fever," an expression used by West Indian slaves to describe the contortions of persons with "breakbone fever." Other theories are that the word comes from *denguero*, Spanish for "affected," or from the Swahili *ki-dinga*, describing a seizure (Haubrich, p. 59).

From the language of Ghana comes *kwashiorkor*. The word means "displaced child," which is probably the social reason behind many children with this severe dietary deficiency, chiefly of protein.

At the beginning of this chapter, I mentioned *mittelschmerz*, from the German words for "middle" and "pain." Mittelschmerz is pelvic pain that occurs at the time of ovulation and that is caused by peritoneal irritation as a response to bleeding from the ovulation site. The pain occurs in the "middle" of the menstrual cycle—midway between the menses, when ovulation occurs.

Tsetse is a word that comes from the language of Botswana, in southern Africa. These bloodsucking African flies of the genus *Glossina* can transmit to humans the trypanosomes that cause the Gambian and Rhodesian forms of African sleeping sickness.

In Japanese, *tsutsugamushi* means "dangerous bug." Scrub typhus is a synonym for tsutsugamushi disease, an acute infectious disease caused by *Orientia tsutsugamushi* and transmitted by chiggers. The disease was found in hemp harvesters in some parts of Japan and is most likely to be found in terrain with secondary (scrub) vegetation.

Yaws is a tropical infectious disease caused by *Treponema pertenue* and is characterized by the development of granulomatous berry-like lesions on the extremities. The name of the disease may have come from an African word for berry (Haubrich, p. 251). Yaws may involve bone, but unlike in syphilis, cardiovascular or central nervous system manifestations do not occur.

Metaphoric Words

A metaphor likens one thing to another, generally alluding to some common characteristic. Many colorful medical words are actually metaphors, which generally make sense when you know the etymologic meaning of the term.

Anthrax, a word used by Hippocrates, is the Greek word for coal (Pepper, p. 120). The allusion may be to the black eschar of the mature lesion or the red-hot appearance of the active lesion.

Today, we use the Latin word for crab—*cancer*—to describe how malignant growths hold tenaciously to the tissues they invade. In another perspective on the metaphor, Haubrich (p. 36) relates this explanation from Galen: "Just as a crab's feet extend from every part of the body, so in this disease (cancer) the veins are distended, forming a similar figure."

The duodenum, from the Latin word *duodecim* (meaning "twelve"), is so named because its length is approximately that of 12 finger widths.

Ichthyosis, a scaling skin condition, comes directly from the Greek word *ichthys*, meaning "fish."

Lens is the Latin word for what we call lentil, a bean often used to make soup. The word was used to describe the major refractive mechanism of the eye because of its similarity in size and shape to the lentil bean.

Lupus, as in lupus erythematosus, comes directly from the Latin word for wolf. The metaphor may refer to the disease's tendency to devour skin or perhaps to the wolf-like appearance of the malar rash.

Some early anatomist observed the bony protuberance of the temporal bone found behind the external ear and concluded that it resembled a woman's breast. That is, it was "breast-like" or *mastoid*. In my youth, the mastoid carried fearful significance. Before the days of antibiotics, middle ear infections could sometimes invade the mastoid sinuses, establishing chronic infection that could be eliminated only by a surgical procedure, a mastoidectomy.

The Latin word for wing is *pinna*, which is the name of the somewhat wing-like external ears found on each side of the head.

Zoster is the Greek word for girdle. In Latin, the word for girdle is *cingulum*. The former was taken directly into our medical vocabulary; the latter entered the medical dictionary as *shingles*. Both describe an eruption that circles the torso, like a girdle that just doesn't cross the midline.

Echoic Words

Echoic words imitate the sound of what they are intended to describe; a more elegant synonym for this phenomenon is *onomatopoeia*. We use these words in everyday speech. Examples are a sudden loud noise (*bang*), the sound made by a cat (*meow*), and the slogan of a breakfast cereal ("Snap, crackle, and pop"). Other familiar echoic words are *beep*, *buzz*, *zap*, *hiss*, *honk*, *mumble*, *pop*, and *whoosh*.

My favorite echoic word is *borborygmus*. A similar word was used in ancient Greece to convey the same meaning as today: elephantine rumbling of the intestines.

Rales comes from the French word *râler*, meaning "to make a rattling sound." The word was introduced to the medical vocabulary by French physician René Laennec (1781–1826), inventor of the stethoscope (in 1816), to describe the lung sounds he heard using his new device (Haubrich, p. 189; Perry, p. 133).

As I look through my word books, I seldom find specific origins for echoic words, as I did for anthrax or tularemia (as described above). Most onomatopoetic words we use seem to have just sprung up. Despite their undistinguished origins, these words make their way into common use because they just make sense.

Below are some other echoic words we use in medicine. Some have antecedents in other languages, but their justification for being in medical English should be apparent:

Burp
Cough
Croup
Hiccup
Murmur
Spit
Whooping cough

Descriptive Phrases

Sometimes, perhaps in a blinding flash of insight, medical terms enter our vocabulary describing just what the phrase denotes in some meaningful, sometimes memorable, and often colorful way.

"Backpacker's diarrhea" is a good example of a descriptive medical phrase. Caused by the flagellated protozoan *Giardia lambia* or *G. intestinalis*, backpacker's diarrhea afflicts naive backpackers who drink untreated water downstream from the sites of defecation of cattle, dogs, rodents, beaver, and even bighorn sheep. Although it carries the sobriquet "backpacker's disease," giardiasis is the most common parasitic infection in the world and America's most prevalent waterborne illness (4).

Shortly after eating in a restaurant serving Asian cuisine, a susceptible person may experience burning in the neck and arms and a sensation of pressure in the chest. The culprit is likely to be monosodium glutamate. Because this compound is commonly used in Chinese cooking, the manifestations are called "the Chinese restaurant syndrome."

"Cotton-mill asthma," aka byssinosis, is an occupationally induced asthma-like disease found in persons who work with cotton, hemp, or flax. The name *byssinosis* comes from the Greek word for flax, *byssos*. Most susceptible are persons working with unprocessed cotton in an enclosed area (that is, in textile mills). The disease has also been called "mill fever," "cotton-dust asthma," and "Monday morning asthma," the latter name reflecting the tendency for the disease to recur when the affected person returned to work.

"Farmer's lung," another occupationally induced disease, is a hypersensitivity pneumonitis caused by inhalation of *Actinomycetes* spores, found in moldy hay. These organisms grow luxuriantly when hay is stored in warm silos and haylofts, and the disease is the most common type of hypersensitivity pneumonitis. It should be distinguished from "silo filler's disease," which is caused by oxides of nitrogen.

When a football player on defense attempts to tackle a runner from behind by grasping his jersey by the fingertips, he risks "jersey finger." The injury is an avulsion of the flexor tendon of the finger which occurs when the full force of a running body overcomes the strength of a small tendon in the hand.

"Little league pitcher's elbow" is a medial epicondylitis sustained by forceful flexion of the wrist/forearm muscles associated with baseball pitching. The recognition of this entity has led to rules limiting the number of pitching innings per week or pitches per game. I once encountered this entity in a young boxer who had a unique style of punching. His technique was to "throw" uppercuts, which (like a baseball pitch) involved the repeated forceful use of the forearm flexors that originate on the medial epicondyle.

An overuse syndrome causing knee pain in persons who jog or run long distances repeatedly is called "runner's knee," or the patellofemoral pain syndrome. It is related to excessive motion of the patella during stride.

"Saturday night palsy" classically occurs in heavy drinkers who fall asleep with one arm draped over the back of a chair or park bench, causing a wrist drop that results from compression of the radial nerve. Some patients have a pre-existing alcoholic neuritis and some do not. A lower extremity variant is a palsy involving the common peroneal nerve as it winds around the proximal fibula, following prolonged sitting up with one leg crossed at the knee and resulting in a foot drop. Both palsies are compression neuropathies that typically resolve spontaneously but may recur if the nerve is subjected to the causative factors described.

"Skier's thumb" and "gamekeeper's thumb" are similar entities, both involving the ulnar collateral ligament. Skier's thumb is an acute injury, a sprain or rupture of the ulnar collateral ligament of the thumb. It occurs when a person falls while holding something, like a ski pole, in the hand and cannot break the fall with the palm of the hand. Instead, the landing is on the thumb, resulting in injury. Gamekeeper's thumb, caused by repetitive injury as the thumb and index finger are used to break the neck of small birds and animals, is seldom encountered today.

World War I brought us two disease nicknames: "trench foot" and "trench mouth." Much of the Great War was fought in deep, water-filled trenches, where soldiers lived and fought for weeks. Trench foot, also called "chilblains" or "immersion foot," describes what happens when feet remain wet and cold, but not necessarily frozen. During World War I, soldiers were provided with whale grease and told to apply it to their feet in an effort to reduce the prevalence of this condition in the trenches. The idea was to make the feet waterproof. In fact, World War I brought trench foot to our awareness, but the disease was described earlier in Napoleon's troops in 1812. A variant seen during the Vietnam War was called "jungle rot." In the U.S., we are most likely to see trench foot in homeless persons exposed to damp, cold conditions.

Trench mouth, properly termed necrotizing ulcerative gingivitis, occurred during World War I when soldiers in the trenches were subjected to unsanitary conditions, poor diet, exposure to the elements, and stress. Folk etymology has attempted to link the term trench mouth to the wooden plates used in medieval times and later—called *trenchers*. Yes, the trencher plates were often wormy and seldom washed, but necrotizing ulcerative gingivitis seems not to have been epidemic at the time, and the term trench mouth (not *trencher* mouth) awaited the circumstances of the Great War.

"Welder's conjunctivitis" is a keratoconjunctivitis induced by ultraviolet irradiation when a welder fails to use adequate eye protection. The same phenomenon occurs in snow conjunctivitis/snow blindness. The Inuit used "goggles" carved from caribou antlers to help prevent snow blindness; most of the rest of us will, we hope, use protective lenses.

New descriptive names are added to our lexicon as physicians connect disease manifestations to activities. In a letter to the *New England Journal of Medicine*, Dahl et al. describe two of these (5). These Alaskan physicians tell of "musher's knee" and "hooker's elbow." Musher's knee is an iliotibial band irritation that leads to lateral knee pain and that is caused by repeated backward kicking of the leg by the team driver at the rear of the sled during "mushing." Hooker's elbow is a lateral epicondylitis that occurs during ice fishing, when the fisher sits at the hole and repeatedly jerks the line upward using a wooden stick. Hooker's elbow is, of course, caused by the same sort of activity as the better-known "tennis elbow."

Confusion, Controversy, and Misadventures in Medical Etymology

Pharyngitis means "inflammation of the throat," *clavicle* comes from a Greek word for key, and "Rocky Mountain Spotted Fever" was first discovered in the Rocky Mountains. If only all medical etymology were quite as logical and straightforward. But sometimes, the evolution of words follows a twisted path, and the original meaning of a word sometimes turns out to be erroneous or misleading. At other times, experts disagree on a word's origin or its place in the lexicographic panoply. Let us look as some of these.

Artery

The word comes from the Latin *arteria*, meaning "windpipe," and from the Greek *aer*, meaning "air." Shipley (p. 290) explains that "since it was noticed that no blood is in them (arteries) after death, it was assumed that the arteries carried air." In his explanation of the body's circulatory system, William Harvey (1578–1657) clarified that arteries carry blood, not air, but the name remained, even though no longer etymologically correct.

Asphyxia

The word for suffocation comes from the Greek roots *a*, meaning "without," and *sphyxis*, indicating "pulse" (Haubrich, p. 22). Of course, following death by suffocation, there is no pulse, nor is their breathing. Today, we use the word to indicate an interference with breathing which, if extreme, will eventually lead to a pulseless state.

Belladonna

We attribute the word *belladonna*, Italian for "beautiful lady," to the wide-eyed, but refractively challenged, Renaissance women who applied the substance to the eyes to enhance their glamour by dilating the pupils. The source of the active compound is the deadly nightshade, a perennial shrub that is highly toxic when ingested. Eating a few berries has poisoned children, but the root of the plant is the most toxic part. Evans IH (p. 98) proposes an intriguing sinister origin for the word *belladonna*, namely that the plant extract was used by an Italian scoundrel named Leucota to poison beautiful women.

Catarrhal Jaundice

Weiss (p. 19) discusses the archaic term *catarrhal jaundice*. In 1864, German pathologist Rudolf Virchow (1821–1902) described mucus plugs in the common bile duct of patients dying of acute liver disease, helping give rise to the term *catarrhal jaundice*, suggesting inflammation of a mucous membrane. Eventually, the disease was found to be infectious hepatitis, hepatitis A, and the term *catarrhal jaundice* now is found only in dusty, outdated medical dictionaries.

Caucasian

If you have been a clinician for more than 20 years, you were probably taught to present a case beginning with something like, "The patient is a 60-year-old Caucasian . . ." Although no longer medically fashionable, the word remains familiar to all of us. Why Caucasian? The Caucasus Mountains in Eurasia near what are now Turkey and Iran and what was once the USSR, where in mythology Zeus chained Prometheus for giving fire to humans, was where a prehistoric skull was discovered. After studying the skull, German scientist Johann Friedrich Blumenbach (1752–1840) proposed the existence of the "Caucasian race," or *Varietas caucasia*. The other families of man were yellow (Mongols), red (American Indians/Native Americans), brown (Malaysians), and black (Ethiopians). The Caucasus region had special significance at the time because of its proximity to Mount Ararat, the landing site of Noah's Ark following the great deluge of biblical times. Because the skull was found in the vicinity of the Ark's landing site, it was logical to conclude that the inhabitants of the region—Caucasians—were the original humans and that any other skin color represented an aberration from the first humans.

Claudication

This medical term comes from the Latin *claudicare*, meaning "to limp." The word reminds us of the fourth emperor of Rome, Claudius I (10 BCE–54 CE), who was the grandson of Mark Anthony and Octavia (sister of Emperor

Augustus) and who is best recalled as the leader who brought Britain into the Roman Empire. Because of some physical disabilities, Claudius I was not a robust young man. Among other afflictions, his knees would not always support him and at times he would fall. Early medical historians held that his disease was probably the result of poliomyelitis. However, poliomyelitis cannot explain all of the known manifestations, such as a shaking head and stammering speech. A current theory is that Claudius I had cerebral palsy. Fast forward to Paris in 1831, when a French veterinarian puzzled over a horse that would trot, then collapse, and then rise only to trot and collapse again. On autopsy, the horse was found to have an obstruction of the femoral artery. Not long after and recalling the affliction of Emperor Claudius I, Sir Benjamin Brody introduced the term *claudication*.

Gonad

The Greek word for seed is *gone*, and from this root we derive our word *gonad*. From this same root comes *gonorrhea*, adding to *gone* the Greek work *rheos*, "to flow." The misconception was that the copious, thick urethral discharge was due to the continuing flow of semen. We now know that the discharge of gonorrhea is caused by purulent material resulting from infection and that it contains no semen at all.

Hypochondriasis

In ancient times, many disorders with obscure origins were attributed to the liver and spleen, housed anatomically under the lower ribs. Hence, one who had a large number of constitutional symptoms came to be called a *hypochondriac* (literally, "under the rib"). Jamieson tells an amusing anecdote about hypochondria. Thomas Sydenham (1624–1629) sent a hypochondriacal patient on a journey to Scotland to consult a learned physician. The patient made the exhausting journey, only to learn that there was no such doctor. He returned to London "full of rage, but cured of his complaint" (6).

Innominate Artery

In writing about the arteries coming from the aorta, Galen (120–200) described but neglected to label one of the main vessels. In the 16th century, the anatomist Vesalius (1514–1564) corrected the deficiency by applying the name *innominate* ("unnamed") *artery*.

Hysteria

This word, which describes a disorder characterized by emotional excitability, comes from the Greek word for womb, *hystera*. In the fifth century BCE, Greek physicians believed that the source of the emotional disorder was the womb, specifically in an aberration in blood flow from the uterus to the brain. From this etiologic misbelief, the logical next step was to name the sensation of a "lump in the throat" or globus hystericus, believing that what the distressed woman felt in her throat was the uterine fundus.

Orthopedic

What does *orthopedics* mean when one examines the word origins? *Ortho* means "straight" in Greek, but what about the other half of the word? It seems logical that the specialty takes it name from the Latin *pes/pedis*, meaning "foot," doesn't it? However, the term, coined in 1741 by Nicholas André (1658–1742) as part of the title of a book, referred originally to straightening the deformities of children. *Paidion* is the Greek word for child.

Mad

When used as a synonym for *insane, mad* is not a popular medical term, but there is an intriguing medical twist, although one that has been questioned. We know the Mad Hatter from Lewis Carroll's *Alice's Adventures in Wonderland.* In Carroll's time, hat makers (or "hatters") sometimes suffered chronic mercury poisoning, as they worked with mercurous chloride in their trade. It seems reasonable to assume that Carroll's connection of *mad* and *hatter* reflected this known occupational hazard. Another explanation, however, is that the phrase predated Carroll, Alice, and hatters. The theory is that the earlier phrase was "mad as an atter." *Atter* was the Anglo-Saxon word for adder, a venomous snake. And in those days, *mad* could mean *insane* or *venomous.* Thus, Carroll's linking the terms *mad* and *hatter* may have been coincidental (7).

Phrenic

The descriptor for phrenic nerve comes from the Greek word *phrēn*, meaning "mind." Think of schizophrenia—a "split mind." It seems that the ancient Greeks used their term for "mind" to identify the muscular diaphragm because emotional turmoil can cause diaphragmatic tightening (Dirckx, p. 67). Although in the fifth century BCE, Hippocrates assured his pupils that the major muscle separating the chest and abdomen lacked mental capabilities, we continue to use the term *phrenic* for structures and function related to the diaphragm.

Western Blot Test

The Western blot test, currently used in the detection of the human immunodeficiency virus (HIV), temporally followed the Southern blot test and the Northern blot test. It would seem that all are named for regions of the United States. Wrong. The Southern blot test was named for the clinician who first described it: Dr. E.M. Southern, who wrote a description of the test in the *Journal of Molecular Biology* in 1975. Next came a somewhat related test, which was named the Northern blot test, simply because the prior test was "Southern." The current Western blot test continues the trend, showing just how playful those research scientists can be.

Etymologic Curiosities in Medicine

Some medical words have come to us by intriguing routes. There is no pattern to these words, which have entered the clinical lexicon in assorted ways:

Since Adam and Eve were our first parents, it seems appropriate to begin this section with the Adam's apple, the laryngeal prominence of the thyroid cartilage which is generally more noticeable in men than in women. Because the Adam's apple is more characteristic of men, transwomen will sometimes seek to have the prominence reduced surgically with a chondrolaryngo-plasty (trachea shave). The 1913 edition of *Webster's Dictionary* attributes the name to the belief that a piece of the forbidden fruit, the apple, became stuck in Adam's throat. There is, however, another theory about the origin of the term. The Latin phrase for the protuberance is *pomum Adami* (apple of Adam). In ancient Hebrew, the laryngeal prominence is called *tappuach ha adam* (male bump), and the subsequent Latin and current English phrases may represent a mistranslation (8).

Atropine comes from Greek roots *a*-, meaning "not," and *tropos*, meaning "to turn." But the tale is more complicated than just a word root with a prefix. The mythological three Fates were the mistresses of destiny. Clotho spun the thread of life, Lachesis measured the thread, and Atropos, generally seen holding the shears of life, made the fateful cut. Once the thread of life was severed, there was no turning back. Atropine, a naturally occurring alkaloid of *Atropa belladonna*, one of the Deadly Nightshade family, is poisonous (see Belladonna above) and thus could cut life's fragile thread.

When I was a child, *bedlam* was one of my mother's pet words, usually evoked when my friends and I were engaged in rambunctious play. Although not in my handy medical dictionary, the word *bedlam* has a medical con-nection. *Bedlam* is a contraction of *Bethlehem*, from the Hebrew word *Beth-lehem*, meaning "house of bread" (Train, p. 13). The Hospital of Saint Mary of Bethlehem was founded in London in 1247 and in 1547 was con-verted into an asylum for "lunatics." The term then evolved to become a metaphor for an insane situation—madhouse.

The *calvarium*, taken directly from the Latin word, is the roof of the skull. Outside the walls of Jerusalem is a hill whose contour gives it the appear-ance of a human skull. The site was called *Golgatha*, "skull hill" in Aramaic. Later, in Latin, it was known as *Calvary*—the place of Christ's crucifixion. "And they took him up to the place Golgotha, which is translated Place of the Skull" (Mark 15:22).

Carotid, the name of large arteries vital to cerebral circulation, comes from the Greek words *karoun* and *karotikos*, meaning "to stupefy or render unconscious." Gershon (p. 2) describes how ancient mystics "attracted an audience by paralyzing a goat with their hands." They pressed on the large arteries in the animal's neck, rendering them unconscious. Galen (120–200) termed the neck vessels *carotikai arteriai*, preserving etymologic integrity. Later, Vesalius (1541–1564) attempted—without success—to rename the arteries (using Latin roots) *soporalis arteriae*, the arteries of sleep (9).

The coccyx, the terminal bone of the spinal column, takes its name from the Greek *kokkyx*, meaning "cuckoo." The Greek physician Herophilos (335–280 BCE), the world's first anatomist, believed the bone resembled the cuckoo's beak.

We can trace the term *condom* to a report about syphilis by Fallopius (1523–1562), although he was probably describing an item that had been in use since long before his time. A popular legend ascribes the word to a Dr. Condom (or some similar spelling), who provided the penile sheaths for King Charles II of England (10). Another tale traces the word *condom* to the 16th century and Pierre de Gondi, the minister of Catherine de Medici and Henry II of France. De Gondi developed waxed sheaths for his patrons, and the French soon adopted the word *gondon* to describe the condom. Variations of *gondon* are used in French and Italian today, and—the elusive Dr. Condom notwithstanding—our word *condom* may be the anglicized version of *gondon*.

Yet another theory holds that the term comes from the village of Condom, in France. It seems that local shepherds used sheep intestines to construct penile sheaths and sold them to travelers. The town of Condom had more travelers than one might expect, because it is situated on one of the French routes of the Way of St. James, followed by pilgrims traveling to Santiago de Compostella in northwest Spain. Eventually, the devices were mailed from France to customers in other countries, being sent in "French letters," a term occasionally used as a synonym for condoms.

Cretinism is no longer used to describe congenital hypothyroidism, perhaps because this once-clinical description found its way into popular use as a pejorative term to describe a person with severe mental retardation (as well as various physical abnormalities). Of a number of sources, only one mentioned the island of Crete, whose inhabitants "were found by venturing Greeks to be completely uninformed of the outside world" (10). Other sources trace *cretin* to an old French word *chrêtien*, meaning "a Christian," and before that to the Latin *creatura*, or "a being." In Romance languages, *Christian* is sometimes used as a synonym for "person." Furthermore, the soil of some areas of the Alps and Pyrenees produces crops that yield a severely iodine-deficient diet. In these areas, "cretinism" is common: the so-called Cretins of the Alps. Thus, Ciardi (p. 92) explains the word *cretin* "with no antireligious sense that Christian faith amounts to idiocy; rather to indicate compassionately a poor deformed creature possessed of a God-given soul and of the grace of baptism."

Delirium comes from the Latin prefix *de-* ("away from") and *lira* ("furrow"). Thus, *delirium* literally means "plowing out of the furrow." I conjure up an image of a confused farmer plowing in a hopelessly crooked line. With delirium tremens in the alcoholic person, the reason for the confusion and wayward plowing can be deduced.

Digitalis, popularized by William Withering (1741–1799) as an extract of the foxglove plant, takes it name from the Latin word *digitus*, meaning "finger." The flower of the foxglove plant has finger-shaped clusters resembling a glove. The "finger" part of the derivation seems straightforward, but how did "fox" become part of the plant name? In 1542, German botanist Leonhard Fuchs (1501–1566) suggested "digitalis" as the plant name, perhaps because the German name for the foxglove plant is *Fingerhut* ("thimble"). Curiously, *Fuchs* is the German word for "fox." All of this 16th and 18th century discovering and naming do not explain another pertinent fact: The plant foxglove has been so called since the 11th century (Haubrich, p. 62).

Fornix comes directly from the Latin word for arch or vault; there are fornices of the conjunctiva, pharynx, stomach, vagina, and uterus. *Fornicate* shares the same root, but with a slightly spicy story. The inhabitants of Rome and Pompeii used arched ceilings in the basement levels of their buildings. These areas often housed the poor and, more to the etymologic point, prostitutes. Thus, the arched areas served as brothels and it was not long before the Latin verb *fornicari* came to mean "to frequent brothels," and from this word comes our current term for sexual intercourse.

Rubella was a recognized disease in Germany and elsewhere for more than two centuries, but it was an American who coined the term "German measles." In 1874, J. Louis Smith at New York's Bellevue Hospital described an outbreak of the disease. Having read reports of similar outbreaks in Germany, he named the disease "German measles" (Bordley and Harvey, p. 657). Because such a disease would have been considered unpatriotic during World War I, it was—quite briefly—called "liberty measles" (Fortuine, p. 250). Does anyone remember "Freedom Fries?"

The mitral valve has its root in the Latin word *mitra*, meaning a "turban." The mitral is a bicuspid valve, and the name connotes its resemblance to a bishop's headdress—the mitre.

Moron is a word coined in the early 1900s by psychologist Henry H. Goddard to indicate an adult with a mental age of 8 to 12 on the Binet scale or an intelligence quotient (IQ) under 51–75. *Moron* was a step up from *imbecile* (IQ of 26–50) and two steps up from *idiot* (IQ of 0–25). This word migrated to common use, with pejorative connotations, and is now a clinical anachronism. What is interesting about the word's origin is this: The root is the Greek *moros*, meaning "stupid" or "foolish." Moron was the name of a dim-witted character in the play *La Princesse d'Elide* by Molière (1622–

1673). Probably both the Greek root and Molière's character were in the minds of members of the American Association for the Study of the Feeble-minded when, in 1910, they voted "moron" into existence, making it one of the very few words ever voted into the English language (Hendrickson, p. 324).

From the Greek word *naus*, meaning "ship," comes our word *nausea*. For many years, this word for this unpleasant symptom was restricted to seasickness; we now use *nausea* in a more expanded context.

Pain comes form Latin *poena*, meaning "penalty" or "punishment." The word's derivation may reflect the Judeo-Christian belief that physical suffering is our punishment for original sin—or perhaps for our own personal sins. The belief in pain as a just punishment was the reason that the development of anesthesia in the 19th century was opposed on religious grounds as antithetical to divine intent.

An abnormal tendency to consume items without nutritional value—clay, ashes, paint, or ice—is called *pica*, which is the Latin word for magpie. These omnivorous birds are known to pick up and store strange objects that are valueless as food.

The "platysma muscle" comes from the Greek word *platys*, meaning "flat or broad." Plato, student of Socrates and founder of the Athenian Academy where Aristotle studied, received his name because of his "broadness," which may have referred to his wide, flat forehead or perhaps to his broad-based wisdom (Gershen, p. 111).

Only one disease is identified by a single letter: Q fever. Why "Q fever"? One theory is that is was named for Queensland, the Australian state where the disease was first identified. Another possibility is this: This disease is not arthropod-borne like other rickettsial infections, and thus its etiology was a mystery for years; the *Q* thus represents the query as to the cause.

Rabies comes from the Latin word *rabere*, "to rage," a symptom that can distinguish dogs and other animals with this acute infectious disease of the central nervous system. The legendary werewolf, a man who turns into a ravenous canine at the time of a full moon, is probably a representation of a rabid animal.

The sacrum was the holy bone: *os sacrum* in Latin. Dirckx (p. 49) explains that the bone gets its name because of "the custom of offering this part of a sacrificial animal on the altar." The aura surrounding this particular bone may be related to a belief that in a decomposing body, the sacrum is the last bone to decay and hence the nidus from which a new body might be formed in the afterlife (Gershen, p. 6).

In Latin, *testis* means "witness." The custom of taking an oath with the hand on one's, or perhaps on someone else's, scrotum began in ancient Greek times. In the Bible we find, "And the servant put his hand under the thigh of Abraham his master, and sware [sic] to him concerning the matter" (Genesis 24:9). Today, testimony, a word derived from *testis*, is preceded by putting one's hand on a Bible, not the male gonad.

Thalassemia, a hereditary hemolytic anemia, comes from Greek words meaning "sea" (*thalassa*) and "blood" (*haima*). The disease is also called "Mediterranean anemia," because it was originally found in persons living near the Mediterranean Sea.

The tragus is a cartilaginous projection of the auricle in front of the external auditory canal. The word means "he-goat" in Greek. This part of the external ear is so named as an allusion to the hairs that grow there, especially in older men, and reminiscent of a goatee.

The vagus nerve takes its name directly from a Latin word meaning "wandering." The vagus nerve meanders on its lengthy anatomical course. Someone who is vague (a word from the same root) wanders discursively in an aimless fashion.

Virus is a Latin word meaning "poison." Only much later did *virus* achieve its current meaning, describing organisms that characteristically (but not always) can pass through fine filters that retain most bacteria and that are unable to grow or reproduce apart from living cells.

References

1. Train J. *Remarkable Words with Astonishing Origins*. New York, NY: Charles N. Potter, Inc.; 1980:9.
2. Butler RF. Sources of the medical vocabulary. *J Med Educ*. 1980;55:128–129.
3. Taylor RB. Please don't call me 'provider.' *Am Fam Physician*. 2001;63:2340–2342.
4. *Entamoeba histolytica* entry. Family Practice Notebook Web site. Available at: http://www.fpnotebook.com/GI99.htm. Accessed August 5, 2006.
5. Dahl W, Matthews K, Midthun J, Sapin P. "Musher's knee" and "hooker's elbow" in the Arctic. *N Engl J Med*. 1981;304:737.
6. Jamieson HC. Men and books; catechism in medical history. *Can Med Assn J*. 1943;48:148.
7. "Mad as a hatter" entry. Urban legends reference pages. Available at: http://www.snopes.com/language/phrases/hatter.htm. Accessed August 5, 2006.
8. MedTerms Medical Dictionary: medical dictionary of popular medical terms. Available at: http://www.medterms.com. Accessed August 6, 2006.
9. Bollet AJ. Medical history in medical terminology, part 2. *Resid Staff Physician*. 1999;45:60–63.
10. "Condom" entry. Web site of Wikipedia, the free encyclopedia. Available at: http://en.wikipedia.org/wiki/Condom. Accessed May 7, 2007.

5
Whose Syndrome? Stories of Medical Eponyms

Which expression would you prefer to use in clinical practice? Myelora-diculopolyneuronitis or Guillain-Barré syndrome? Type VII mucopolysaccharidosis or Sly syndrome? Frontotemporal lobar degeneration or Pick disease? If you chose the former in each case, you belong to the growing legion of antieponymists. If you prefer the latter choices, you are an old-fashioned eponym fancier.

The word *eponym* can mean a person (or place or event) for which something is named or can describe the word so derived. Bloomers were named for American feminist Amelia Bloomer (1818–1894), the Bunsen burner takes its name from Professor R.W. Bunsen (1811–1899), and Morse code was created by American inventor Samuel Morse (1791–1872) (Fowler, p. 160). In medicine, Addison disease (chronic adrenocortical insufficiency) was first described by British physician Thomas Addison in his 1855 publication *On the Constitutional and Local Effects of Disease of the Suprarenal Capsules*. Thus, Dr. Addison is the eponym for the disease. Those who have Addison disease are often referred to as "Addisonian," and hence the word *Addisonian* may also be called an eponymous word. Body parts, diseases, syndromes, drugs, microorganisms, and more may all have eponymous origins.

Naming things after those associated with their origins is a time-honored academic tradition. Consider the honorific names Osler disease (polycythemia vera) and Weber-Christian syndrome (relapsing febrile nodular nonsuppurative panniculitis). The definitive work on eponyms is Jablonski's *Illustrated Dictionary of Eponymic Syndromes, and Diseases, and Their Synonyms*, listing some 9,000 medical eponyms (1).

Today, there is an increasing bias against the use of medical eponyms. Perhaps it is elitism, scientific purism, or some sort of egalitarian political correctness. Here are some of the arguments against eponyms. To begin on a humorous note, August Bier (1861–1949) asserted that, "When a disease is named after some author, it is very likely that we don't know much about it" (Strauss, p. 116). Whether or not that statement is true, there is certainly room for confusion with some eponyms. For example, Addison disease of the adrenal gland, mentioned above, must not be confused with Addison anemia (pernicious anemia).

In fact, the campaign against the use of eponyms is hardly new. More than a century ago, in 1903, Richards wrote of the "evils of eponyms," decrying especially the then-popular tendency to "associate methods of treatment, and especially operations, with the names of their real or supposed originators, and to describe them under the heading of this or that person's operation or method of treatment" (2). As examples, the author cited the Caldwell-Luc operation, Killian's operation, and the Rinne test.

As in life itself, there is not always fairness in eponyms. The name of English surgeon Sir James Paget (1814–1899) is attached to a cell, a stain, a disease, and a syndrome. Sir Jonathan Hutchinson (1828–1913) is the eponymous ancestor of eight anatomic abnormalities, a syndrome, and a disease. Whereas dozens of otherwise obscure physicians will be recalled by posterity by managing to have their name attached to some arcane biochemical abnormality, William Harvey (1578–1657), who in 1628 first described the circulation of blood, has not a single eponym to his name.

Ravitch has an even more jaundiced view of eponyms, holding that most eponyms will have one or more of the following deficiencies: The eponym fails to honor the original describer, the honored person failed to understand or did not recognize the significance of the discovery, the currently used term does not reflect the original concept, and the attribution lacks historical basis in the first place (3).

The above notwithstanding, I am a fan of eponyms. I believe that our medical understanding and, indeed, our lives are enriched as we consider the historical antecedents of the fallopian tube, the circle of Willis, tetralogy of Fallot, and Wegener granulomatosis.

There is a current trend to omit the possessive 's from eponyms. Thus, Reiter's syndrome has become Reiter syndrome. I have no objection to the deviation from tradition. After all, German bacteriologist Hans Reiter (1881–1969) may have described the triad of urethritis, iritis, and arthritis, but he did not "own" it. Throughout this chapter, I have eliminated the terminal possessive.

Honorific Names of Diseases, Syndromes, Treatment Methods, and More

Here, in more or less chronological order, are some noteworthy eponyms. I have necessarily made choices among the 9,000 eponyms in our panoply, giving a special nod to those associated with our heroes described in chapter 1.

The Greek "Father of Medicine," Hippocrates (ca. 460–377 BCE), lends his name to a host of eponymous words and phrases: The **hippocratic facies** of the moribund person, the **hippocratic fingers** and **hippocratic nails** also called "clubbing," the **hippocratic wreath** of hair characteristic of male-pattern baldness, and **hippocratic succussion**, a splashing sound produced by shaking the torso when there is gas or air and fluid in the body cavity. There is also the **Hippocratic Oath**, mentioned in chapter 1.

Andreas Vesalius (1514–1564), the Flemish anatomist who became Professor of Anatomy at the medical school in Padua, is honored by several eponymous structures—all appropriately anatomical. The **Vesalius bone**, or *os vesalianum*, is a tuberosity of the fifth metatarsal bone which at times occurs as a separate bone. The **Vesalian vein** passes through the **foramen of Vesalius** or sphenoidal emissary foramen. Fortuine (p. 270) describes the **ligament of Vesalius** as a synonym for the inguinal ligament, but I could not confirm this term in my current editions of *Dorland's Illustrated Medical Dictionary* or *Stedman's Electronic Medical Dictionary*.

The first person to describe and illustrate the cerebral circulation was English physician Thomas Willis (1621–1675), in his 1664 book *Cerebri Anatome*. We know the cerebral arterial loop as the **circle of Willis**. Today, medical students dutifully memorize the names of the branches arising from this arterial circle.

Sydenham chorea is named for Thomas Sydenham (1624–1689), who described the syndrome in his book *Schedula Monitoria*, published three years before his death. Sydenham chorea describes involuntary spasmodic movements sometimes found following a streptococcal infection and in conjunction with acute rheumatic fever.

The troika of goiter, hyperthyroidism, and often exophthalmos was described in 1786 by English physician Caleb Parry (1755–1822), later in 1802 by Italian physician Giuseppe Flajani (1741–1808), and then by Robert Graves (1797–1853) in Ireland in 1835, and subsequently by Karl von Basedow (1799–1854) in Germany in 1840. Here is the significance of this chronology: In Germany, the disease is called **Basedow disease**, in Italy it is **Flajani disease**, and in the English-speaking world we use the term **Graves disease**. Note the terminal *s* without the possessive in using the name Graves. *Stedman's Electronic Medical Dictionary* still lists **Parry disease** as a synonym for Graves disease.

We, quite appropriately, immortalize Louis Pasteur (1822–1895) with the eponymous **pasteurization**, the use of heat to kill harmful microorganisms. The process, first tested in 1862, does not aim to eliminate all organisms from the food or beverage. (Do you recall Pasteur's "Beer of Revenge" in chapter 1?) Rather, the process achieves a "log reduction" in the population of viable organisms, reducing the risk of disease—assuming proper refrigeration and reasonably prompt consumption. There is also the **Pasteur vaccine** for rabies and the bacterial genus formerly named *Pasteurella*, which included *P. pestis* (plague) and *P. tularensis* (tularemia). *P. pestis* is now termed *Yersinia pestis*; *P. tularensis* is now *Francisella tularensis*. Microbiologists are quite fond of changing names of microorganisms to honor more modern scientists, to the great consternation of us humble clinicians who struggle to keep current with the scientific names of organisms that cause the diseases we see.

The syndrome of motor and vocal tics transmitted in an autosomal dominant pattern is called **Tourette syndrome**. It is named for French physician Georges Gilles de la Tourette (1857–1904), who was a student of neurologist Jean-Martin Charcot (1825–1893) in Paris. Some patients who have Tourette syndrome also have coprolalia, from the Greek *kopros*, meaning "dung," and *lalia*, signifying "talk." Fortuine reports that Tourette's index patient in 1895 was a French woman whose illness included the coprolalia manifestation. "When she died at the age of 85, the Parisian newspapers were pleased to quote some of her more salacious utterances" (Fortuine, p. 307).

German physicist Wilhelm Roentgen (1845–1923), who discovered x-rays in 1895, has had his name scattered widely across the radiologic landscape. We have **Roentgen rays** and **units**. There are **roentgenograms**, **roentgenography**, **roentgenometers**, and **roentgenoscopes**. Some patients receive **roentgenotherapy**, now termed radiotherapy.

Sir William Osler (1849–1919), physician educator and medical author, has lent his name to a number of entities. These include the **Osler nodes** (small, erythematous skin lesions seen in patients with subacute bacterial endocarditis), **Osler disease** (polycythemia vera, also known as **Osler-Vaquez disease**), and **Rendu-Osler-Weber syndrome** (hereditary hemorrhagic telangiectasia).

The **Gram stain**, or **Gram's method**, is a technique of staining microscopic slides, allowing the microscopist to differentiate between two groups of bacteria, based on staining characteristics. The two groups are broadly defined as gram-positive or gram-negative organisms. The method was invented by Danish biologist Hans Christian Gram (1853–1938). Pepper (p. 92) describes a rumor, which he concedes is "probably untrue." Legend holds that Gram first observed the differential staining after accidentally spilling a bottle of iodine over a slide he was preparing. Even if the discovery was serendipitous, at least Gram recognized its significance and potential utility.

Also known as oculo-oral-genital syndrome or malignant aphthosis, **Behçet syndrome** was named for Turkish dermatologist Hulusi Behçet (1889–1948), who first described a triad of manifestations: ocular uveitis, oral aphthous ulcers, and genital ulcers. Dr. Behçet noted that three of his patients had similar symptoms, which might represent a previously unrecognized disease, which he described in a paper published in 1937 in the journal *Dermatologische Wohenschrift*.

In 1959, as a Temple Medical School student doing a clinical rotation at St. Christopher's Hospital in Philadelphia, I observed several members of a family that possessed curious characteristics. These individuals each had one or more of the following: impaired hearing, prematurely gray hair, and different-colored eyes; each had a noticeable white forelock. My attending physician correctly identified these patients as having **Waardenburg**

syndrome, named for Dutch ophthalmologist Petrus Johannes Waardenburg (1886–1979), who presented a case at a medical meeting in 1947 and published an account of this case the next year. Thus, in retrospect, the family that I encountered as a medical student had a disease that, at that time, had been recognized for little more than a decade. Over the past 50 years, I have looked in vain for my next patient with Waardenburg syndrome.

In 1952, American anesthesiologist Dr. Virginia Apgar, practicing in New York City, devised a five-criteria scoring system to assess the well-being of newborn infants. The **Apgar score** criteria—skin color, heart rate, reflex irritability, muscle tone, and respiration—were each assessed on a scale of 0, 1, or 2. A total of 10 was a perfect score, indicating a robust newborn. More than a decade later, in 1963, pediatrician Joseph Butterfield linked the five criteria to the five letters in Dr. Apgar's name. The eponym thus also became an acronym: **A**ppearance, **P**ulse, **G**rimace, **A**ctivity, and **R**espiration. The "grimace" was a bit of a stretch, but the memory device has helped medical students recall the scale ever since. Of course, things did not stop there. In Spanish, the words are *Apariencia*, *Pulso*, *Gesticulatión*, *Actividad*, and *Respiración*. In German, the acronym becomes *Atmung*, *Puls*, *Grundtonus* (probably a better fit than "grimace"), *Aussehen*, and *Reflexe*. Then, in 1978, Smilkstein proposed the Family APGAR as a test to evaluate family function. Using the widespread clinical familiarity with the eponymous Apgar test, Smilkstein proposed to evaluate family function by assessing five components: **A**daptation, **P**artnership, **G**rowth, **A**ffection, and **R**esolve (4). In 1990, I paid a visit to some young physicians in Quito, Ecuador. One of the questions they asked was, "Dr. Taylor, can you explain the Family APGAR test and how to use it in practice?" Dr. Apgar never received the Nobel Prize, but she was pictured on a United States 20-cent postal stamp in 1994.

Five Eponymous Diseases Likely to Endure

Some diseases closely allied to individuals seem likely to survive the efforts to purge eponyms from our medical vocabulary. Here are some of them:

Munchausen Syndrome

Munchausen syndrome has other names. One is the tomomania syndrome, from the Greek words *tomos*, meaning "to cut," and *mania*, or "frenzy." The patient with Munchausen disease may also be called a "peregrinating problem patient," from the Latin *peregrinus*, "to wander." Through several phases of etymologic evolution, the Latin *peregrinus* became our word *pilgrim*, although we still retain the word *peregrinate*, meaning "to travel," in our English language dictionaries.

Munchausen patients wander from doctor's office to emergency room to surgical clinic—offering an often-astonishing variety of complaints that classically suggest problems that have operative remedies. The presentation may be hemoptysis or perhaps blood in the urine. The Munchausen patient knows how to produce the blood-containing specimen when needed. Abdominal pain occurs commonly, and these persons will submit to extensive diagnostic testing and sometimes exploratory surgery.

Who was Munchausen? The syndrome is named for Karl Friedrich Hieronymus, the Baron von Münchhausen (note the slight spelling variation), a German officer who had served with the Russian cavalry in the 1739 war against the Ottoman Turks. During his retirement years, he told tall tales of his military experiences and other exploits.

In 1785, Rudolf Erich Raspe in England published a book entitled *Baron Munchausen's Narrative of His Marvellous Travels and Campaigns in Russia*, more or less attributed to the stories of the real Baron, who by then was retired in the small town of Bodenwerder, Germany. Raspe changed the spelling of his hero's name to Munchausen, which is the spelling that has been attached to the clinical syndrome. Raspe, it seems, was eventually charged with an instance of fraud and fled to avoid imprisonment, leaving us to wonder about the attribution and veracity of his writings.

No connection between the real and the fictitious barons and anything clinical was made until 1951, when British physician Sir Richard Asher (1912–1969) proposed the eponymic descriptor for the complex mental illness (5).

Pickwickian Syndrome

Mr. Pickwick, although rotund, did not have pulmonary alveolar hypoventilation associated with corpulence, which we now call **Pickwickian syndrome**. In the Charles Dickens novel *The Posthumous Papers of the Pickwick Club* (aka *The Pickwick Papers*), published in 1837, Mr. Wardle's servant boy, Joe, is both extremely obese and afflicted with a tendency to fall asleep while performing everyday chores:

"Damn that boy," said the old gentleman, "he's gone to sleep again."
"Very extraordinary boy, that," said Mr. Pickwick, "does he always sleep in this way?"
"Sleep!" said the old gentleman, "he's always asleep. Goes on errands fast asleep, and snores as he waits at table."
"How very odd!" said Mr. Pickwick.

Although Dickens described the "fat boy" in 1837, the medical link awaited the turn of he century. Fortuine (p. 265) tells us that the first clinician to liken an overweight, somnolent youth to Mr. Wardle's boy Joe was Sir William Osler (1849–1919). According to this author, in 1906 Osler described, "an extraordinary phenomenon associated with excessive fat in young persons [to be] an uncontrollable tendency to sleep—like the fat boy in Pickwick." (Fortuine does not provide the reference citation, and I have been unable to locate it.) Today, we have an **O**xford **SLE**ep **R**esistance test, eponymously termed the OSLER test, to assess daytime sleepiness.

Apparently, the simile did not catch on. If so, we might have yet another eponymous syndrome associated with Sir William's name and not merely a slightly contrived test name. Instead, credit for popularizing the term pickwickian syndrome goes to Bicklemann et al., who in 1956 reported the case of a 51-year-old executive who suffered obesity, fatigue, and somnolence. The authors cite an example of the significance of the patient's inappropriate sleepiness. "The patient was accustomed to playing poker once a week and on this crucial occasion he was dealt a hand of three aces and two kings. According to Hoyle this hand is called a 'full house.' Because he had dropped off to sleep he failed to take advantage of this opportunity. A few days later he entered ... hospital" (6). I grieve that we no longer see such memorable depictions of disease manifestations in current medical writing.

My first encounter with Pickwickian syndrome is deeply etched in my memory. It occurred in 1959, three years after the condition was named. The venue was, once again, St. Christopher's Hospital for Children in Philadelphia, and I was a third-year medical student. Into the emergency room came a 12-year-old boy, extremely obese, dyspneic, and hypoxic. The child promptly went into cardiac arrest; closed cardiac compression on the very overweight chest was futile, and the courageous resident made a large surgical incision and I participated in my first open cardiac massage.

Down Syndrome

The eponym **Down syndrome** will probably still be used a generation or two from now because it is nonjudgmental and easier to remember than trisomy 21. Down syndrome is not uncommon, occurring in about 1 in 800 to 1,000 live births. Patients with Down syndrome have a recognizable countenance, and because they can often lead productive lives, we see them often in the community. Noteworthy persons with Down syndrome include actors Stephane Ginnsz in the Martin Scorsese film *Duo*, Chris Burke in the television series *Life Goes On*, and singer Miguel Tomasin, with the Argentinian band Reynols.

The syndrome, which combines impaired learning ability and growth with characteristic facial features, was described in 1846 by Edward Séguin (1812–1880) as "furfuraceous idiocy." *Furfuraceous* comes from a Latin word meaning "scaly," as is seen in dandruff. Children with Down syndrome often have rough, dry skin, which may be why Séguin chose this term. The "idiocy" label was unfortunate, because it stuck until the 20th century.

The next chapter in the story is the tale of British physician John Langdon Down (1828–1896). Early in his medical career, Down was appointed to the post of superintendent of the Royal Earlswood Asylum for Idiots in Surrey. Down seems to have been a very capable superintendent, and in his clinical work he set out to describe the disorders found in his institution's residents. He used photographs to study patients with the same constellation of findings. Down suggested that the features "might be a throwback to the Mongol racial type" (Porter, p. 587). From that time, **mongolian idiocy** was the generally accepted term until 1961, when a panel of geneticists pleaded with *The Lancet* for a better term, suggesting four alternatives. The journal editor chose Down's syndrome, now Down syndrome, and the name seems destined to endure (7).

Parkinson Disease

James Parkinson (1755–1824), a student of John Hunter, called the disease paralysis agitans in his 1817 *Essay on the Shaking Palsy*, in which he described the characteristic tremor, gait, and other features of the disease. We tend to think of medical heroes as one-dimensional, but this is generally erroneous. For example, Parkinson reported the first case of appendicitis described in English. He also was a paleontologist who wrote treatises on fossils and a political activist who authored controversial pamphlets (Garrison, p. 424).

Parkinson's work on paralysis agitans was followed by that of Jean-Martin Charcot, who was the one to coin the term **Parkinson's disease** (Porter, p. 547).

Although we have recognized and studied parkinsonism for almost 200 years, there are currently no laboratory tests that can detect the disease, and the diagnosis continues to be clinical—based on a medical history and physical examination. The finding that only 75% of clinical diagnoses are substantiated by autopsy results supports the view that the disease, at least in its early stages, is difficult to diagnose with certainty (8).

Public interest in a disease, often expressed as research funding, increases when famous persons are affected, especially if there are recognizable manifestations. Noteworthy Parkinson disease sufferers have included artist Salvador Dali, evangelist Billy Graham, and Pope John Paul II. The disease afflicted dictators Francisco Franco, Adolf Hitler, and Mao Zedong. A type of parkinsonism has struck boxers such as Muhammad Ali (formerly Cassius Clay) in later life. The film *Awakenings*, starring Robert De Niro, dealt with postencephalitic parkinsonism and helped heighten awareness of neurologic diseases in general. Recently, actor Michael J. Fox, who developed parkinsonism at a young age, established a foundation for research, with the aim of finding a cure for the disease.

Alzheimer Disease

If we look in the scientific literature, we find several papers published in German in 1906 and 1907 by Alois Alzheimer (1864–1915), a neuropathologist who did his most important work in Munich in conjunction with Emil Kraepelin (1856–1926), the "Linnaeus of Psychiatry." In fact, Kraepelin, as a clinician, was the first to identify the characteristic manifestations of memory loss and forgetfulness as well as the behavioral changes, disinhibition, and disorientation. Alzheimer was a neuropathologist who had published a six-volume *Histologic and Histopathologic Studies of the Cerebral Cortex*, with stunning illustrations. Working with Kraepelin, Alzheimer sought to understand the neuropathology behind the disease manifestations.

Alzheimer's index case was a 51-year-old woman who suffered progressive illness with dementia leading to death at the end of five years. At autopsy, Alzheimer used silver staining techniques to demonstrate clumping of neurofibrils in her cerebral cortex (Beighton and Beighton, p. 9).

As their findings became clearer, Kraepelin, in a gesture that must stand as unique in the history of medical scholarship, decided to step aside from the naming of the disease they had co-discovered and allowed the single name Alzheimer to become the eponym. One theory is that Kraepelin wished to focus attention on the neuropathologic origins of mental disorders.

Kraepelin would go on to describe dementia praecox, which he defined as the "sub-acute development of a peculiar simple condition of mental weakness occurring at a youthful age" and which Eugene Bleuler (1857–1940) later renamed schizophrenia.

Until the 1970s, **Alzheimer disease** meant "presenile dementia" in persons ages 45–65. As we came to know more about the disease, the "pre" was dropped, and the term now denotes primary senile dementia. Alzheimer disease causes 70 percent of all dementia and is the fourth leading cause of death in the United States.

With hundreds of millions of dollars devoted to Alzheimer disease research each year, and in the absence of a handy scientific name, the eponymous term appears here to stay.

More About Eponyms

Eponymic Diseases, Syndromes, and Drugs

Cesarean Section

The first word in this section may not be a true eponym at all, and it represents an example of uncertain—even disputed—etymology. We clinicians often think of the term **cesarean section** as describing how young Julius (100-44 BCE) entered the world through an incision into the uterus via the mother's abdominal wall. But there are some flaws in the story. Pepper (p. 170) writes that in the days of the Caesars, hysterotomy to save the baby was done only if and when the pregnant woman died and that, "Abdominal extraction was not done on the living mother until the sixteenth century."

That said, what about the presumably eponymous word *cesarean*? The word probably comes from the Latin word *caesus*, meaning "the cut one." The cognomen was already well established in the Julian line of the family Caesar at the time of little Julius' birth, perhaps because some distant ancestor was delivered by a "caesarean" birth (Ciardi, p. 54).

Ondine's Curse

There is no question about the eponymous origin of **Ondine's curse**, describing the hypothalamic alveolar hypoventilation syndrome, a rare condition causing apnea owing to the loss of automatic control of respiration (9). Ondine, aka Undine, was a water nymph in German mythology. The nymph married a mortal, Sir Lawrence, who pledged that his "every waking breath shall be my pledge of love and faithfulness to you." When Sir Lawrence inevitably proved unfaithful, Ondine cursed him with an affliction that reprised his pledge to her: He could breathe voluntarily while awake, but he would die if he should fall asleep. In time, sleep overtook him and, lacking automatic respiratory activity, he died of suffocation. Ondine was discussed in the writings of Paracelsus, and the nymph is the antecedent for an opera by E.T.A. Hoffman, a piano movement by Ravel, a play by Jean Giraudoux, an asteroid, and a U.S. Navy ship.

Nicotine

The namesake for our word **nicotine** was Jean Nicot (1530–1600). Nicot was the French ambassador to the royal court at Lisbon. When tobacco plantings were brought from the New World, Nicot cultivated them and introduced the noxious weed to Europe in 1560. When Swedish botanist and zoologist Carolus Linnaeus (1707–1778), the "Father of Modern Taxonomy," classified nature into a hierarchy in the 18th century, he named the genus of the plant *Nicotiana*. The specific compound nicotine was later isolated and named in 1819.

Listerine

Here, we recall Lord Joseph Lister (1827–1912) from chapter 1. In 1866, Lister used carbolic acid (phenol) to help achieve sterile surgical technique. Although most scientists feel honored by eponymic immortality, Lister was not at all pleased when *Listerine* was formulated and marketed during his lifetime.

Dr. Joseph Lawrence and Jordan Wheat Lambert developed the product in 1879. First used as a surgical antiseptic (as Lister had used carbolic acid), the product was later marketed to dentists and then as an over-the-counter mouthwash. It was touted to "kill germs that cause bad breath," a phrase that I find to be a coy use of words. Note the direct absence of a claim that it stops bad breath. The ingredients in Listerine are eucalyptol, thymol, menthol, methyl salicylate, and, of course, an alcohol concentration exceeding 20 percent. Note the total absence of Dr. Lister's carbolic acid/phenol.

Dirckx (p. 82) reports that Lister "spent vast sums of money in unsuccessful efforts to suppress the term, which seemed to link him with a product that had no connection with him or his work."

Huntington Chorea

The story of eponymous **Huntington chorea**, also called **Huntington disease**, began when a young man spent time with his physician father. American physician George S. Huntington (1850–1916) was a third-generation small-town physician on Long Island, New York. Huntington described in a 1909 lecture how, as a youth, he first became interested in the disease that bears his name:

"Over 50 years ago, in riding with my father on his rounds I saw my first case of 'the disorder,' which was the way the natives always referred to the dreaded disease. I recall it as vividly as though it had occurred but yesterday. It made a most enduring impression on my boyish mind, an impression which was the very first impulse to my choosing chorea as my virgin contribution to medical lore. Driving with my father through a wooded road leading from East Hampton to Amagansett we suddenly came upon two women bowing, twisting, and grimacing. I stared in wonderment, almost in fear. What could it mean? My father paused to speak to them and we passed on. Then my Gamaliel-like instruction began; my medical instruction had its inception. From this point on my interest in the disease has never wholly ceased" (10).

As an aside, Gamaliel was a renowned rabbinical scholar of biblical times, sometimes said to have been a teacher of St. Paul.

In a remarkable feat of epidemiological excavation, Huntington demonstrated that the disease could be traced to a mutant gene carried to the U.S. in 1830 by immigrants from a small village in Suffolk County, England (Cartwright, p. 171). At least one author believes that the affected family came to America on the *Mayflower* (Fortuine, p. 307). Cartwright also states that, "The violent twitching and mental symptoms aroused suspicion and caused some of those affected to be accused in the notorious Salem witch trials in 1692" (p. 171). (This explanation conflicts with the theory that the Salem witch hallucinations were induced by ergot derivatives; see chapter 3.)

Sir William Osler (1849–1919) gave his imprimatur to the eponymy when he wrote, "In the history of medicine there are few instances in which a disease has been more accurately, more graphically or more briefly described" (11).

Because the disease caused the disability and death of famous folk singer Woody Guthrie, Huntington chorea will be mentioned again in chapter 9.

Sister Mary Joseph Node

This eponym honors Sister Mary Joseph Dempsey (1856–1939), first surgical assistant to Dr. William Mayo (1861–1939) and nursing supervisor at Saint Mary's Hospital in Rochester, Minnesota. As surgical assistant, Sister Mary Joseph would prep the abdomen of patients prior to surgery. From time to time, she would note an enlarged node in the periumbilical area, generally indicating metastasis from a gastric carcinoma and consequently a grim prognosis. Her observation led this finding to be called the **Sister Mary Joseph node**.

Hallervorden-Spatz Syndrome

This eponym describes neurodegeneration with brain iron accumulation type 1. The disease is a rare, inherited dystonic disorder that would be otherwise forgettable except for the fate of the eponym. Because of alleged euthanasia of mentally ill patients during World War II, the names of the two doctors previously associated with the disease have been purged, and the descriptive scientific name now prevails.

Patients Immortalized in Eponyms

Not many diseases are named for patients. Physicians and scientists seem to prefer to attach their own names, not those of the patients, to discoveries. We have already mentioned pickwickian syndrome and Munchausen syndrome; although both are named for persons, neither is precisely linked to a real human being. Here are some conditions in which the naming is more specific.

Pott Fracture

The eponym denotes a bimalleolar fracture involving the lower part of the fibula and the malleolus of the tibia, with lateral displacement of the foot. British surgeon Percival Pott (1713–1788) has a special claim on the Pott fracture because he was the index case. Pott sustained the bimalleolar fracture when he fell from a horse and, in 1750, wrote an account of his fracture. We also remember Pott for his 1779 description of Pott disease, tuberculosis of the spine with kyphosis, and several other eponymic abnormalities.

Hunterian Chancre

The primary lesion of syphilis is sometimes named for a famous patient—Scottish surgeon John Hunter (1728–1793)—who himself had syphilis. I will tell you the full story of one of medicine's classic misadventures in chapter 11.

Mortimer Disease

In 1898, Jonathan Hutchinson (1828–1913) described a patchy dermatitis that affected one of his patients, identified as "Mrs. Mortimer" (12). The term Mortimer disease, sometimes employed in the past as a synonym for Boeck sarcoid or sarcoidosis, is seldom used today. Hutchinson, however, achieved considerable eponymic fame; in current use, we find the Hutchinson crescentic notch, facies, freckle, incisors, mask, patch, pupil, teeth, and triad. It is too bad that Mrs. Mortimer's eponym has fallen into obscurity.

Christmas Disease

Christmas Disease, also known as hemophilia B, is a genetically transmitted clotting disorder involving factor IX. It takes its name from Stephen Christmas, youngest of the seven patients described in the initial report of the disease. The paper, by Dr. Rosemary Biggs, was published in the *British Medical Journal* in 1952. The paper appeared that year in the December (think *Christmas*) issue (13).

Hartnup Disease

Also described in the 1950s was Hartnup disease, a genetic metabolic disorder of tryptophan absorption in which the chief manifestation is a scaly, red rash and photosensitivity. The disease was first noted in a London family named Hartnup.

Daltonism

My *Stedman's Electronic Medical Dictionary* lists daltonism as a synonym for a color vision deficiency, especially deuteranomaly or deuteranopia. The defect was named for English physicist John Dalton (1766–1844), whose legendary colorblindness resulted in his occasionally wearing attire "whose hues scandalized his fellow Quakers" (Dirckx, p. 82).

Legionnaires Disease

This disease is named for a large group of patients. Note the lack of possessive in the term. A century from now, will anyone recall that Legionnaires disease was first described when it struck 221 veterans attending the 58th Annual Convention of the Pennsylvania American Legion and others staying at the historic Bellevue-Stratford Hotel in Philadelphia in the summer of 1976? Thirty-four of the affected persons died. The hotel was soon forced to close but has since re-opened with lodging on the upper floors. A decade or so later, exhibiting great courage, I stayed in this remodeled hotel and can report that I suffered no ill effects.

Lou Gehrig Disease

The classic example of modern patient-oriented eponym construction is Lou Gehrig disease, amyotrophic lateral sclerosis. This inevitably fatal neurodegenerative disease has also been called Aran-Duchenne disease and Charcot disease, but the English-speaking world will recall it as Lou Gehrig disease long after the legendary athletic achievements of the namesake are forgotten. Henry Louis (Lou) Gehrig (1903–1941) played Major League Baseball for the New York Yankees. His astounding record of playing in 2,130 consecutive games ended with the progression of his neurologic disorder. The record for consecutive games played endured until bested by Cal Ripkin, Jr., of the Baltimore Orioles in 1995. Gehrig was inducted into the Baseball Hall of Fame in 1939, two years before he died of his disease.

Eponyms With Intriguing Origins

Job's syndrome takes its name from the biblical character, whose body was covered with boils by Satan. The disease is a rarely occurring hyperimmunoglobulin E syndrome that causes staphylococcal skin infections, among its other manifestations.

Literary allusions have given us some memorable eponyms. From *Gulliver's Travels*, published in 1726 by Jonathan Swift (1667–1745) as a thinly disguised political satire, comes **Lilliputian syndrome**, a hallucinatory state in which the person sees people and objects as tinier than they actually are. From the fertile mind of Lewis Carroll (1832–1898), author of *Alice's Adventures in Wonderland*, come several medical allusions. **Humpty-Dumpty syndrome** describes a tendency to attribute a wide variety of health and other problems to a single memorable event. In **Alice in Wonderland syndrome**, the individual experiences visual and perceptual disturbances; I will return to this syndrome in chapter 9.

Another eponym based on literature is **Jekyll and Hyde syndrome**, sometimes called dissociative identity disorder or bipolar behavior. In his novella, the *Strange Case of Dr. Jekyll and Mr. Hyde*, Scottish author Robert Louis Stevenson (1850–1894) described a terrifying example of bipolar behavior and provided an early model of the psychological thriller. There is a story that, while writing the book, Stevenson was being treated with an ergot derivative, which I described in chapter 3 as sometimes causing psychoactive disturbances. Could there be a pharmaceutical link to the literary inspiration, as perhaps there was with Lewis Carroll?

Whereas some eponyms come from literary characters, others arise from the names of authors. Two of these authors have seen their names joined in the lexicon of psychopathology: **Sadism** comes from the name of Marquis de Sade (1740–1817), a French count and novelist whose works contained detailed descriptions of sexual perversions. To him is attributed the quotation, "Sex without pain is like food without taste." From the Austrian author

Leopold Ritter von Sacher-Masoch (1836–1895), whose best-known work is entitled *Venus in Furs*, comes the word **masochism**, denoting a perversion—often sexual—in which a person takes pleasure in being mistreated and humiliated.

Another somewhat morbid eponym is **Van Gogh syndrome**, named for Dutch artist Vincent van Gogh (1853–1890). On Christmas Eve in 1888, van Gogh cut off his ear with a razor after a heated quarrel with his colleague Paul Gauguin. Following this incident, van Gogh spent much time in mental hospitals before his death by self-inflicted gunshot wound in 1890. Since that time, the disturbed tendency to self-mutilation has borne his name.

Some eponyms introduced over recent years seem to be a little over-reaching. Nevertheless, here they are: **Rapunzel syndrome**, reported in 1968, describes the long strands of hair extending from a bezoar in the stomach through the intestine (Magalini, p. 451). Mandibular prognathism is sometimes called **Hapsburg jaw**, referring to a facial feature found in many members of the Hispano-Austrian imperial dynasty. **Popeye syndrome** occurs in persons, such as drummers, whose forearm muscles become hypertrophied, making the forearms larger than the upper arms. Sometimes, when performing histologic diagnosis of a thyroid tumor, the pathologist encounters enlarged cells with "ground glass" nuclei called **Orphan Annie eye nuclei**, a finding that suggests malignancy. The lip damage sometimes seen in trumpet players is called **Satchmo's syndrome.** The restless leg syndrome has been called **Fred Astaire legs**. Do not bother looking for any of these in the medical dictionary.

C.K. Tashima, an America physician who proudly (and with tongue in cheek) named a syndrome for himself, described my favorite eponym. **Tashima syndrome** describes a condition in which a physician searches earnestly for a new symptom, sign, syndrome, or disease to which to attach his or her own name (14).

References

1. Jablonski S. *Illustrated Dictionary of Eponymic Syndromes, and Diseases, and Their Synonyms*. Philadelphia, PA: Saunders; 1969.
2. Richards GL. The evils of eponyms. *JAMA*. 1903;41:893–894.
3. Ravitch MM. Eponyms. *Med Times*. 1968;96:1149–1151.
4. Smilkstein G. The family APGAR: a proposal for a family function test and its use by physicians. *J Fam Pract*. 1978;6:1231–1239.
5. Asher R. Munchausen's syndrome. *Lancet*. 1951;1:339–341.
6. Bickelmann AG, Burwell CS, Robin ED, Whaley RD. Extreme obesity associated with alveolar hypoventilation; a Pickwickian syndrome. *Am J Med*. 1956;21:811–818.
7. Ward OC. John Langdon Down: the man and the message. *Downs Syndr Res Pract*. 1999;6:19–24.
8. Gelb D, Oliver E, Gilman S. Diagnostic criteria for Parkinson disease. *Arch Neurol*. 1999;56:33–39.

9. Deonna T, Arczynska W, Torrado A. Congenital failure of automatic ventilation (Ondine's curse). A case report. *J Pediatr.* 1974;84:710–714.

10. Huntington G. Recollections of Huntington's chorea as I saw it at East Hampton, Long Island during my boyhood. *J Nerv Ment Dis.* 1910;37:255–257.

11. Osler W. Historical note on hereditary chorea. *Neurographs.* 1908;1:113–115.

12. Hutchinson J. Cases of Mortimer's malady (lupus vulgaris multiplex non-ulcerans et non-serpiginosus). *Arch Surgery London.* 1898;9:307–314.

13. Biggs R, Douglas AS, MacFarlane RG, Dacie JV, Pitney WR, Merskey C. Christmas disease: a condition previously mistaken for haemophilia. *Br Med J.* 1952;2:1378–1382.

14. Tashima CK. Tashima's syndrome. *JAMA.* 1965;194:208.

6
Medical Abbreviations, Acronyms, Euphemisms, Jargon, and Slang

Medical scientific terms are the meat and potatoes of clinical discourse. Abbreviations, acronyms, euphemisms, jargon, and slang are the condiments. They add flavor to what might otherwise be multi-syllabic discussions. These sometimes arcane, occasionally insightful, communication tools allow us to convey information in a shorthand manner, often in ways unintelligible to the non-medical person, at least so we think.

Abbreviations

In *medicalese*, an ELF is not a strange little man in green tights; the term refers to elective low forceps or to endoscopic laser foraminotomy. PET is positive electron tomography, not a domesticated animal. SPA is not where one goes for a relaxing massage; it stands for serum prothrombin activity (or one of nine other possibilities).

This chapter is not intended to be useful in a clinical sense. It is not the place to go when pondering the meaning of PNSP (penicillin-nonsusceptible *Streptococcus pneumoniae*) or BOU (burning on urination). The clinically helpful book on abbreviations (ABRs) is *Medical Abbreviations*, by Neil M. Davis, currently in its 13th edition (1). Davis insightfully subtitles his book *28,000 Conveniences at the Expense of Communication and Safety*. This section is for enrichment, to help us understand the context and scope of medical abbreviations.

I begin with the method used by medical writers to create abbreviations. In the previous paragraph, I created an abbreviation for the word "abbreviation"—ABR. (This abbreviation is not in Dr. Davis' latest book, but perhaps he will include it in the 14th edition.) Now, by custom, for the remainder of the chapter I can use either the full word "abbreviation" or the shorthand ABR that I have created.

This all works very well when a chapter or an article is short and when there are not too many ABRs. Reading becomes tiresome when the author uses many unfamiliar ABRs whose solitary explanations are scattered throughout pages of text. Consider the following sentence from a published chapter on obstetric complications: "UCs in the presence of a positive FFN triples the risk of PTB." This sent me scrambling to confirm that UCs meant uterine contractions, FFN is fetal fibronectin, and PTB stands for pre-term birth.

Commonly Used Medical Abbreviations

Disease Abbreviations

There are many abbreviations used to indicate the names of diseases or abnormalities. Just a few of them are:

Abbreviation	Disease
ALL	Acute lymphocytic leukemia
BPH	Benign prostatic hypertrophy
COPD	Chronic obstructive pulmonary disease
MS	Multiple sclerosis
PDA	Patent ductus arteriosus
RA	Rheumatoid arthritis
SLE	Systemic lupus erythematosus
URI	Upper respiratory infection

Diagnosis and Treatment Abbreviations

The following is a list of some time-tested, generally accepted medical abbreviations in regard to clinical diagnosis, laboratory testing, and treatment which every physician and nurse should know.

Abbreviation	Meaning
ACTH	Adrenocorticotropic hormone
ALT	Alanine aminotransferase (serum glutamic pyruvic transaminase, or SGPT)
ANA	Antinuclear antibody
AST	Aspartate aminotransferase (serum glutamic oxaloacetic transaminase, or SGOT)
b.i.d.	Twice a day (*bis in die*)
BP	Blood pressure
BS	Blood sugar
BUN	Blood urea nitrogen
CBC	Complete blood count
Cl^-	Chloride
CO_2	Carbon dioxide
CPR	Cardiopulmonary resuscitation
CSF	Cerebrospinal fluid

Abbreviation	Meaning
CT	Computed tomography
cu. mm.	Cubic millimeter
CXR	Chest x-ray
d	Day, daily
dL	Deciliter
DM	Diabetes mellitus
ECG	Electrocardiogram
ESR	Erythrocyte sedimentation rate
FDA	U.S. Food and Drug Administration
g	Gram
GI	Gastrointestinal
Hbg	Hemoglobin
Hg	Mercury
HIV	Human immunodeficiency virus
HMO	Health maintenance organization
hr	Hour
h.s.	Hour of sleep, at bedtime
HTN	Hypertension
IM	Intramuscular
INR	International normalized ratio
IU	International unit
IV	Intravenous
K^+	Potassium
kg	Kilogram
L	Liter
LD or LDH	Lactate dehydrogenase
mEq	Milliequivalent
mg	Milligram
min	Minute
mL	Milliliter
mm	Millimeter
mm^3	Cubic millimeter
MRI	Magnetic resonance imaging
Na^+	Sodium
NSAID	Non-steroidal anti-inflammatory drug
p.o.	By mouth (*per os*)
PT	Prothrombin time
PTT	Partial thromboplastin time
q	Every
q.i.d.	Four times a day (*quater in die*)
q.o.d.	Every other day (*quaque altera die*)
RBC	Red blood cell
SC	Subcutaneous

Abbreviation	Meaning
sec	Second
STD	Sexually transmitted disease
t.i.d.	Three times a day (*ter in die*)
TSH	Thyroid-stimulating hormone
U	Unit
UA	Urine analysis
WBC	White blood cell, white blood count
μg	Microgram

Abbreviations With Several Possible Meanings

Far too many abbreviations have a wide range of possible meanings. When using these, the author must be sure to identify what the abbreviation is meant to represent. Otherwise, we might think that a patient with mitral insufficiency (MI) has a myocardial infarction or someone needing tender loving care (TLC) might be counseled on a therapeutic lifestyle change.

Here are just a few examples of ABRs with multiple meanings:

Abbreviation	Possible Meanings
CA	Canceled appointment
	Cancer or Carcinoma
	Candida albicans
	Cardiac arrest
	Carotid artery
	Chronological age
	Community-acquired
	Coronary artery
	Coronary angioplasty
NP	Nasal prongs
	Nasopharyngeal
	Near point
	Neuropsychiatric
	Not palpable
	Not performed
	Not present
	Nursed poorly
	Nurse practitioner
PE	Pedal edema
	Pelvic examination
	Physical examination
	Plasma exchange
	Pulmonary edema
	Pulmonary embolism

Abbreviations That Might Be Hazardous to the Patient's Health

Recently, one of our physicians told the following true story: "I wrote a prescription for a pregnant patient that read, 'PNV one qd #QS x 9 months.' Luckily, the pharmacist called to ask me, 'What dose of Penicillin V do you want?' I explained that I had meant prenatal vitamins." Some abbreviations are easy to misread or misunderstand and can be downright perilous. I recommend that the following abbreviations disappear into the ether of lexicographic history. Most are used in lists of hospital orders, sometimes still handwritten even in the age of electronic medical records, and subject to misunderstanding even when the letters are written clearly.

Abbreviation	Possible Misunderstanding: ABR could be read as . . .
au (ear)	o.u. (each eye)
D/C (discharge)	DC (discontinue)
IU (international unit)	IV (intravenous)
o.d. (once daily)	Right eye
q.d. (daily)	q.i.d. (four times a day)
q. h.s. (every bedtime)	q. h. (every hour)
q.n. (every night)	q. h. (every hour)
U (unit)	0 (i.e., zero, causing a 10-fold increase in a dose)
x3d (three days?)	Or does the order mean "times three doses?"
μg (microgram)	mg (milligram)

Clinicians should generally avoid abbreviations for names of drugs. For example, does MP stand for "melphalan and prednisone" or for "mercaptopurine?" When the nurse carries out an order for the patient to receive AZT, will the drug be zidovudine or azathioprine? Does "nitro" mean nitroglycerin or nitroprusside?

I also recommend that we no longer use:

Apothecary symbols, generally not taught in medical or nursing schools today
Roman numerals, which are no longer readily understood
The virgule (or the slash mark, /) anywhere in writing drug doses; this symbol can be misread as the number 1 and lead to a dangerous dosing error.

As we prepare to leave the topic of abbreviations, I want to discuss the origins of some symbols we use as abbreviations. The symbol ♂ for male comes from the spear and shield of Mars, the Roman god of war; the symbol ♀ for female represents the hand mirror of Aphrodite, Greek goddess of beauty.

The Rx symbol comes from an Egyptian pictogram representing the "eye of Horus," the god of the sun, often represented as a falcon or a man with the head of a falcon. Another theory is that the symbol comes from the Latin word *recipe*, meaning "to take." This symbol served as the prototype for a number of similar abbreviations: Cx for cervix, Dx for diagnosis, Fx for fracture, and Hx for history.

Acronyms

Acronyms, also known as initialisms, are more fun than abbreviations because of the inventiveness involved in constructing them. The word *acronym* comes from the Greek *akros*, meaning "tip," and *nym*, meaning "name." Although scholars claim a few ancient examples exist, acronyms are a relatively new linguistic phenomenon for the most part. They are not unique to medicine. A popular acronym is LASER, the letters representing Light Amplification by Stimulated Emission of Radiation. The military is the source of many of our widely used acronyms. AWOL, meaning "absent without leave," was coined during World War I. The military has also given us WAC (Women's Army Corps), SONAR (Sound Navigation And Ranging), RADAR (RAdio Detection And Ranging), and SNAFU (Situation Normal, All Fouled Up).

Over the years, the concept of acronyms has expanded to connote a term that can be *pronounced* as a word. Thus, we do not say S-C-U-B-A; instead, we say "scuba" to indicate "self-contained underwater breathing apparatus." This tendency to develop pronounceable acronyms has let to the gradual insertion of these manufactured words into our vocabulary. In the years to come, how many persons will recall that SONAR, OPEC, and even AIDS began as acronyms?

Medical Acronyms That Are Sometimes Helpful

Medical acronyms, like abbreviations, can speed up communication and are especially useful when they help us recall or understand a complicated set of facts. Some can be traced to their original authors, most cannot. Here are some examples:

The PRICE syndrome describes the acute treatment of contusions and sprains: Protection, Rest, Ice, Compression, and Elevation.

CABG, pronounced "cabbage," describes a Coronary Artery Bypass Graft. TURP stands for TransUrethral Resection of the Prostate, and gastrointestinal reflux disease is GERD. Both TURP and GERD are pronounced as we would expect from the spelling.

The CAGE questions, devised by Ewing, describe four queries to help detect alcoholism. The key words in the questions regarding alcohol use are Cutting down, Annoyed by criticism, feeling Guilty, and taking a morning

Eye-opener (2). Today, most senior medical students can describe the handy CAGE questions. Another measure of alcohol use disorders is the Alcohol Use Disorders Identification Test (AUDIT) (3).

Some pregnant patients with preeclampsia-eclampsia develop the HELLP syndrome—Hemolysis, Elevated Liver enzymes, Low Platelets.

The acronym ELISA describes a type of laboratory test, and the word comes from Enzyme-Linked Immunosorbent Assay. Note that "assay" means test and thus to speak of an "ELISA test" is redundant.

PANDAS indicates Pediatric Autoimmune Neurologic Disorder Associated with Streptococcal infection.

Organophosphate poisoning can cause the SLUD syndrome: Salivation, Lacrimation, Urination, and Diarrhea.

Here are some more commonly encountered clinical acronyms:

Acronym	What the Acronym Represents
ACE (inhibitors)	Angiotensin-Converting Enzyme
COX	CycloOXygenase
CREST (syndrome)	Calcinosis, Raynaud phenomenon, Esophageal dysmotility, Sclerodactyly and Telangiectasia
DMARD	Disease-Modifying Anti-Rheumatic Drug
Echovirus	EnteroCytopathic Human Orphans + Virus
PEEP	Positive-End Expiratory Pressure
SAD	Seasonal Affective Disorder
SOAP	Subjective, Objective, Assessment, Plan
STAR (complex)	Sore throat, Temperature elevated, Arthritis, and Rash (seen in some viral infections, such as rubella)

Even in medicine, the U.S. government is a rich source of acronyms. OHSA (pronounced "O-sha") is the Occupational Safety and Health Administration, CLIA stands for the Clinical Laboratory Improvement Amendments of 1988, and HIPAA is the Health Insurance Portability and Accountability Act of 1996.

Clinical Trials and Acronyms

There seems to be an unwritten rule that a clinical trial needs a catchy acronym. I am not sure where the trend started but today almost every published study seems to have a cleverly devised title. Stanbrook et al. looked at 173 consecutive randomized trials published between 1953 and 2003 from all systemic reviews completed by the Cochrane Heart Group as of January 31, 2004. Of the 173 studies reviewed, one third had acronymic names. What is even more intriguing, the authors found that randomized clinical trials with acronyms were cited twice as often as those not named with acronyms (4).

Here are some clinical trials with witty acronyms. A few of these are a bit over-reaching and seem to represent "backronyms"—starting with an acronym and finding words to fit the letters:

Clinical Trial Name	What the Acronym Represents
ALLHAT	Antihypertensive and Lipid Lowering Treatment to Prevent Heart Attack
CAPRICORN	Carvedilol Post Infarct Survival Control in Left Ventricular Dysfunction
CHARM	Candesartan in Heart Failure Assessment of Reduction in Mortality and Morbidity Trial
COPERNICUS	Carvedilol Prospective Randomized Cumulative Survey
EPHESUS	Eplerenone Heart Failure Efficacy and Survival Study
PAPABEAR	Prophylactic Oral Amiodarone for the Prevention of Arrhythmias That Begin Early After Revascularization, Valve Replacement, or Repair
PROGRESS	Perindopril Protection Against Recurrent Stroke Study
RALES	Randomized Aldactone Evaluation Study

Acronymic Medical Argot

It is with great misgivings that I write the following short section on acronymic words used to conceal meaning or convey humor, especially in a book that mentions our honored heroes such as Hippocrates, Sydenham, and Osler. But, in fact, medical argot is part of medical heritage and culture, and the book would be incomplete without some mention of these words.

Acronymic medical argot sometimes arises when young clinicians are faced with the combination of long hours, intense work, demanding superiors, and sometimes even more demanding patients. At times, what they encounter is depressing, unclean, and downright grizzly. The construction and use of acronymic slang may provide some small measure of emotional self-defense. Some of the terms that follow are, frankly, derogatory, but they exist in our hospitals and clinics.

GOK stands for "God only knows" and is often the best diagnosis one can offer when confronted with a complex case. A less well-known variation is UBI, unexplained beer injury. FLK, pronounced "flick," indicates a funny-looking kid, often one with a chromosomal abnormality. And when all else fails, there is TEETH—"tried everything else, try homeopathy."

Shem's novel *The House of God* describes the GOMER—derived from the phrase "Get Out of My Emergency Room." Shem describes a GOMER as "a human being who has lost—often through age—what goes into being a human being" (5). Shem also describes the LOL in NAD, the little old lady in no acute distress.

IGBO is a useful acronym for how we, as individuals, sometimes make clinical decisions. The letters stand for "I got burned once," connoting that when you or I have experienced an unfortunate outcome in the past, it influences how we handle the problem in the future. A classic example would be a young woman with what seems to be a small breast lump. If in the past you encountered just such a presentation and it turned out to be invasive cancer, the experience influences your approach from then on.

Today, we have far more clinical guidelines than we can recall or even find readily. Not all of them are spectacularly useful, and the wise clinician checks to see how a particular guideline was created. The best guidelines are based on a solid foundation of randomized clinical trials. The least reliable are considered to be GOBSAT guidelines—Good Old Boys Sat Around a Table.

I will list some more acronymic slang and abbreviations below.

Acronymic Argot	Meaning
GRAFOB	Grim Reaper At Foot Of Bed
HIBGIA	Had It Before, Got It Again
HIVI	Husband Is Village Idiot
LOLITS	Little Old Lady In Tennis Shoes
MARP	Mind-Altering Recreational Pharmaceutical
SIO	Sleeping It Off
TOBP	Tired Of Being Pregnant (often seen near the end of gestation)
UNIVAC	Unusually Nasty Infection, Vultures Are Circling
VIP	Very Intoxicated Person

I will list some non-acronymic slang later in the chapter when I discuss euphemisms, jargon, and slang.

Acronyms as Medical Mnemonics

Medical mnemonics—memory devices—have helped many of us who have trouble remembering lists. In fact, one might say that generations of young physicians have elevated mnemonics to an art form. I learned my first medical mnemonics in anatomy class during my freshman year of medical school. Actually, I didn't learn them "in class," because our professors, who always seemed to be blessed with total recall of obscure details, seldom taught mnemonics. Mnemonics were shared, passed from one student to the next like secret messages, as ways to remember the names of the 12 cranial nerves or the five structures found in the groin. Today, mnemonics seem to be gaining some respectability. For example, first-year medical students in our medical school are taught in their physical diagnosis classes some of the memory devices I once learned from classmates, as well as some that did not exist during my medical school years.

The word *mnemonic* is derived from the name of the Greek goddess of memory, Mnemosyne, whose notable achievement was that, following a tryst with Zeus, she became the mother of nine offspring—the nine Muses.

Although most medical mnemonics are acronyms, a few are actually acrostics. The latter term comes from the Greek *akros*, "tip" or "outermost", and *stichos*, "line of verse." An acrostic is a composition, usually a poem, in which the first letter or syllable of each line spells out another message. In a sense, these are meta-acronyms. The medical school mnemonic I recall most clearly is an acrostic:

> On Old Olympus' Towering Tops
> A Fin and German Viewed Some Hops

The words in the ditty are cues to the names of the 12 cranial nerves:

Word from Poem	Cranial Nerve
On	1. Olfactory
Old	2. Optic
Olympus	3. Oculomotor
Towering	4. Trochlear
Tops	5. Trigeminal
A	6. Abducens
Fin	7. Facial
And	8. Acoustic
German	9. Glossopharyngeal
Viewed	10. Vagus
Some	11. Spinal accessory
Hops	12. Hypoglossal

And now that you can recall the names of the cranial nerves, the following will help tell which are sensory (S), motor (M), or both (B):

> Some Say Marry Money,
> But My Brother Says Big Breasts Matter More.

Here is another acrostic, which helps us recall the names of the carpal bones:

> Scared Lovers Try Positions
> That They Can't Handle.

The first letters of each word are cues to the bone names: scaphoid, lunate, triquetrum, pisiform, trapezium, trapezoid, capitate, and hamate.

Here is an especially clever meta-acronym, in which a few word clues provide more than just initial letters. It tells the names of the tarsal bones:

> Connie Couldn't Count Cubes,
> Never Tackled Calculus.

The names of the bones are first cuneiform, second cuneiform, third cuneiform, cuboid, navicular, talus, calcaneus.

On a humorous note, when trying to recall the branches of the external carotid artery, medical students think: Some Anatomists Like Flirting, Others Prefer S & M. The first letters of these words indicate arterial branches: Superior thyroid, Ascending pharyngeal, Lingual, Facial, Occipital, Posterior auricular, Superficial temporal, and Maxillary.

Finally, here is an anatomic mnemonic that had nothing to do with me, even thought it bears my name. A medical student first told it to me. The brachial plexus has Roots, Trunks, Divisions, Cords, and then Branches. Recall these structures with the acronym: Robert Taylor Drinks Cold Beer.

Anatomic Acronymic Mnemonics

The anatomy dissection room is filled with mnemonics, although they generally lack the poetic lilt of those listed above. Most are simple acronyms. The ones that endure, however, have a definite flair. Here is a sample:

The acronym for the names of the muscles of mastication is BITEM: Buccinator, Internal pterygoid, Temporalis, External pterygoid, and Masseter.

The radial nerve innervates BEST: the Brachioradialis, Extensor, Supinator, and Triceps muscles.

NAVEL helps name the inguinal structures, from lateral to medial: Nerve, Artery, Vein, Empty space, and Lymphatic.

In my physical diagnosis class, students learn the locations on the chest where they can best hear the various heart sounds: the Aortic, Pulmonic, Tricuspid, and Mitral areas. Students can choose among three handy acronyms: APT. M; Al Pacino, The Man; and one I learned recently, again from a medical student, Always Party 'Til Morning.

Acronymic Mnemonics in Clinical Practice

We use a large number of memory devices in daily practice. Those that help in diagnosis seem to predominate. A classic, familiar to many of today's medical students, gives clues to the many possible causes of disease: The acronym is VINDICATE. The letters stand for:

> Vascular causes
> Inflammatory or Infectious disease
> Neoplastic disorders
> Degenerative or Deficiency states
> Intoxication

Congenital causes
Autoimmune or Allergic disease
Trauma
Endocrine (or metabolic) disorders

When evaluating physical pain, think PAIN: Period (duration) of the pain, Area of the pain, Intensity of pain, and Nullify—that is, what makes it go away. Parenthetically, what is missing here is the question: What makes the pain worse?

When pondering the cause of an electrocardiographic ST elevation, use the mnemonic ELEVATION. The letters represent:

Electrolyte causes
Left bundle branch block
Early repolarization
Ventricular hypertrophy
Aneurysm
Treatment, such as a recent pericardiocentesis
Injury, including acute myocardial infarction or contusion
Osborne waves (hypothermia)
Non-occlusive vasospasm

An enlarged spleen may have one of six causes, suggested by the acronym SPLEEN:

Sequestration (e.g., hereditary spherocytosis)
Proliferation (e.g., malaria, infectious mononucleosis)
Lipid disorder (e.g., Gaucher or Niemann-Pick disease)
Engorgement (e.g., portal hypertension or traumatic hemorrhage)
Endowment (e.g., congenital hemangioma)
iNfiltration (e.g., lymphoma, granulomatous disease).

MEDIAN TRAP suggests causes of the carpal tunnel syndrome: Myxedema, Edema, Diabetes mellitus, Idiopathic inflammation, Amyloid disease, and Neoplasm such as a ganglion, Trauma, Rheumatoid arthritis, Acromegaly, and Pregnancy.

The characteristics of a melanoma include Asymmetry, Border irregularity, Color variation, Diameter greater than 6 mm, and Elevation: ABCDE.

I like the mnemonic for the differential diagnosis of right lower quadrant pain: APPENDICITIS: Appendicitis/abscess, Pelvic inflammatory disease or Period, Pancreatitis, Ectopic pregnancy or Endometriosis, Neoplasia, Diverticulitis, Intussusception, Cyst of ovary, Inflammatory bowel disease, Torsion of the ovary, Irritable bowel syndrome, and Stone in the kidney or even the gall bladder.

Many of our medical students know SIGECAPS, pronounceable as a "word," but otherwise meaningless—except that it helps recall the characteristics of depression:

Sleep disturbance, either difficulty sleeping or hypersomnia
Interest in usual activities is diminished.
Guilt feelings or sense of worthlessness
Energy level is decreased.
Concentration is poor.
Appetite changes, either decrease or increase
Psychomotor manifestations
Suicidal ideation

A memorable acronym telling the possible causes of transient urinary incontinence is DIAPPERS. The letters in the acronym stand for Delirium/confusion, Infection of the urinary tract, Atrophy of vagina/urethra, Pharmaceuticals, Psychologic causes, Excessive excretion as with diabetes mellitus or heart failure, Restricted mobility, and Stool impaction.

Surgeons know the five *W*'s of post-operative fever:

Wind: atelectasis or pneumonia
Wound infection
Water: urinary tract infection
Walking: connotes that lack of postoperative ambulation can
    predispose to venous thromboembolism
Wonder drugs: anesthesia complications

HELPER-R helps us to recall the management of shoulder dystocia during an obstetrical delivery. The letters in the acronym stand for Help (request urgently), Episiotomy, Legs flexed and abducted, Pressure in suprapubic area, Enter vagina (to rotate shoulder), Roll the patient onto all fours, and Remove the posterior arm (6).

As the last item in this section of the chapter and to honor the Renaissance anatomist Vesalius, I present the mnemonic for the causes of low back pain: O, VESALIUS. The letters represent: Osteomyelitis, Vertebral fracture, Extraspinal tumors, Spondylolisthesis, Ankylosing spondylitis, Lumbar disc disease, Intraspinal tumors, Unhappiness (depression or malingering), and Strain (Bloomfield and Chandler, p. 94).

Medical Euphemisms, Jargon, and Descriptive Slang

In this section, I will tell a little about some agents of circumlocution—words that can soften, disguise, and sometimes obfuscate the blunt facts of disease and health care.

Euphemisms

In earlier times, we used euphemisms to protect sensibilities. For example, in Victorian times, childbirth was not discussed in polite company, and we therefore used more delicate terms such as "confinement." Today, we still see the abbreviation, EDC, or Estimated Date of Confinement, to indicate the anticipated day of obstetrical delivery. Dirckx tells us that the syphilitic chancre was called a "specific ulcer" and gonorrhea was called "specific urethritis," the latter term offering insight into our current phrase nonspecific urethritis, indicating urethritis that is not due to *Neisseria gonorrhoeae* (Dirckx, p. 31).

Today, we say that laboratory animals are "sacrificed" rather than killed. Venereal diseases are still sometimes called "social diseases." We use the word "stool" awkwardly to describe the normal function of defecation. A woman may be termed "unwell" during her menses, as if she had some sort of disease. Persons with severe handicaps are "physically challenged." The word "disease" is itself a euphemism, coming from words meaning "without comfort."

"Therapeutic substitution" or even "step therapy" describes the act in which the pharmacist or insurance company dispenses a less expensive drug instead of the one prescribed by the physician. A person who abuses drugs is "chemically dependent." These persons and others with potentially expensive chronic diseases may be "deselected" by a health insurance plan.

If the doctor has a "misadventure" during a medical procedure, it may result in an "adverse event." An older individual may have "old-timer's disease" when we don't want to specify primary senile dementia or Alzheimer disease. A fatal disease is sometimes described as "incompatible with life."

Medical Jargon and Descriptive Slang

There is a thin line between medical jargon and slang, and I will consider them together. Both represent an informal vocabulary, and the chief difference seems to be that jargon is somewhat more respectable, while slang is more unrefined. Sometimes it is difficult to tell the difference.

In an effort—sometimes futile—to discuss a disease without the patient understanding what we are saying, we sometimes use oblique terms, such as *lues*, an outdated term for syphilis; *heme*, when we want to discuss blood; and *ethanolism*, to describe chronic alcohol abuse.

If a patient has a very unusual tumor, he or she has a "fascinoma." You thought you saw a problem on an x-ray, but the radiologist did not confirm your finding; what you saw was a "hallucinoma." If the problem is considered to be imaginary—all in the patient's head—we say it is "supratentorial." On the other hand, he or she may be sent to the operating room to be "surgerized."

If there is an infection justifying antimicrobial therapy, we say that the patient has an "antibiotic deficiency." The clinician may then prescribe a very potent antibiotic—a "gorillacillin." When we want to discuss the evaluation of a suspected hypochondriacal patient, the laboratory tests may include a fictitious "serum porcelain level," derived from the practice of labeling such patients "crocks." If someone at the end of life dies, he or she may be "transferred to the eternal care unit."

Here are some other examples of medical jargon and slang:

Term	What it Means
Babygram	A roentgenogram of the entire body of an infant
Departure lounge	Geriatric ward
Donorcycle	Motorcycle, whose riders sometimes become organ donors
Dusting and cleaning	Dilatation and curettage
GI rounds	A clinician's meal or a snack, typically consumed in the hospital cafeteria
Goat rodeo	An emergency setting when nothing goes right
House red	Blood
Knife and gun club	An emergency room in a rough neighborhood
O sign	Patient asleep with mouth open
Parentectomy	Removing one or both parents from the examination room or hospital bedside
Pharmaceutically enhanced	Strongly medicated or "stoned" personality
Q sign	O sign, with tongue hanging out
Sieve	A resident physician who seems to admit every patient encountered
Slow code	A resuscitation effort performed without urgency on a patient whose time to die has come, but the family or the chief of service seem to think otherwise
Soft admission	A patient a Sieve will admit, but a Wall would not
Train wreck	A case in which one complication follows another
Turf	A verb meaning to refer a patient to another specialty service
Virgin abdomen	A patient who has never has abdominal surgery
Wall	The opposite of a Sieve, who is skillful at preventing Soft Admissions to the hospital
Zebra	A very unusual disease, discussed in chapter 7 (aphorisms)

Physicians sometimes poke fun at other specialties and sometimes even at themselves. (For example: How do you hide a dollar bill from an orthopedist? Answer: Put it in a book. How do you hide it from an abdominal surgeon? Tape it over the patient's chest.) Here are some slang terms for various medical specialists:

Slang Term	**Medical Specialty/Specialist**
Baby catcher	Obstetrician
Cath jockey	Invasive cardiologist
Flea	Internal medicine specialists
Gas passer	Anesthesiologist
Headshrinker ("shrink")	Psychiatrist
Knuckle dragger	Orthopedist
Pediatron	Pediatrician
Rear admiral	Proctologist
Slasher	Surgeon
Stream team	Urologists
Unclear medicine	Nuclear medicine

References

1. Davis NM. *Medical Abbreviations: 28,000 Conveniences at the Expense of Communication and Safety.* 13th ed. Huntington Valley, PA: Neil M. Davis Associates; 2006.
2. Ewing JA. Detecting alcoholism. The CAGE questionnaire. *JAMA.* 1984;252: 1905–1907.
3. U.S. Department of Health and Human Services. *Assessing Alcohol Problem Use.* Rockville, MD: U.S. Department of Health and Human Services; 1995: series 4:11,22,260. National Institutes of Health publication 95–3745.
4. Stanbrook MB, Austin PC, Redelmeier DA. Acronym-named randomized trials in medicine–the ART in medicine study. *N Engl J Med.* 2006;355:101–102.
5. Shem S. *The House of God.* New York, NY: Dell; 1978.
6. Carlan SJ, Angel JL, Knuppel RA. Shoulder dystocia. *Am Fam Physician.* 1991;43:1307–1311.

7
Medical Aphorisms

Since the days of Hippocrates, our father, the aphorism has been the literary vehicle of the doctor... Laymen have stolen the trick from time to time, but the aphorism remains the undisputed contribution of the doctor to literature.

Howard Fabing and Ray Marr, in *Fischerisms* (1)

In my first year of medical school, we had a lecture by a surgeon. This was a treat for freshman medical students in the late 1950s—to have a talk by a real doctor, one who actually saw patients. The surgeon began the much-anticipated lecture by writing on the blackboard, in very large letters: *"Primum non nocere!"* This was my first medical aphorism. Of course, I wondered at the time why he couldn't have written "First, do no harm" in English, especially since—as I will discuss below—the saying is frequently attributed to Hippocrates, who lived on the island of Kos, spoke Greek, and probably didn't know Latin at all.

About Aphorisms

Aphorisms, Maxims, Proverbs, and Epigrams

An **aphorism** is a terse, often witty statement denoting a general truth. It is concise, thoughtful, and often based on the author's personal observations. The word *aphorism* comes from the Greek word *aphorismos*, "a pithy sentence." Medicine's claim on the aphorism is valid, because the literary device was used in the *Aphorisms* of Hippocrates, which begins with the well-known saying: "Life is short; art is long; opportunity fleeting; experience perilous; and decision difficult" (2,3). Although various translations differ slightly, the saying and others like it have style, elegance, and longevity. Aphorisms are undoubtedly the aristocrats of medical writing.

You can recognize a good clinical aphorism. It is something you want to share with students and even tell to your husband or wife. You resonate with the saying's lyrical quality and sometimes you can even envision a metaphorical image. For example, consider the following, written by Jean-Martin Charcot (1825–1893), of Charcot joint and triad fame: "Symptoms, then, are in reality nothing but the cry of tormented organs." Can you picture the tears and feel the discomfort of the beleaguered body part?

I hold that an aphorism is invariably attributable to a specific person and that in the long history of medical writing no timeless aphorism was ever penned by a *team* of writers.

Fowler's *Dictionary of Modern English Usage* lists **maxim** as a synonym for aphorism (p. 31). The word *maxim* comes from the Latin *maxima*, as in *maxima proposito*—"the greatest premise." On a historical note, the same entry describes **gnome** as a synonym for aphorism which is no longer used.

A **proverb**, from Latin words meaning "forth" (as in "put forth") and "word," is also a concise saying, generally one that has come to enjoy common use. Spanish writer Miguel de Cervantes states, "Proverbs are short sentences drawn from long experience," a saying which—in itself—may qualify for maxim or proverb status.

Epigram is another word for a concise saying, often one that is witty or satirical. However, because of its origin from the Greek word *epigraphein*, meaning "to write on," I suggest that the word connotes something written. I began the chapter with an epigram written by Fabing and Marr in their monograph cataloging the aphorisms of scientist Martin H. Fischer (1879–1962). In the text quoted, Fabing and Marr describe how "laymen have stolen the trick from time to time" (1). In fact, non-professionals have penned some enduring aphorisms, health-related and otherwise. Just a few of them are presented here:

"An ounce of prevention is worth a pound of cure." (Benjamin Franklin, American statesman)
"A hungry dog hunts best." (Lee Trevino, American golfer)
"Better to remain silent and be thought a fool, than to open your mouth and remove all doubt." (Mark Twain, American writer)
"Genius is one percent inspiration and ninety-nine percent perspiration." (Thomas A. Edison, American inventor)
"He who goes to the law holds a wolf by the tail." (Robert Burton, English churchman and scholar)

If after reading this chapter, you would like to read more about aphorisms in general, I recommend Geary's *The World in a Phrase: A Brief History of the Aphorism* (4). In this book, the author proposes five rules for a proper aphorism. To qualify as an aphorism, a saying must be brief, be definitive, be personal, have a twist, and be philosophical.

The sayings cited in the rest of this chapter may or may not—in your opinion—fulfill all of Geary's criteria; they are presented for your personal enrichment, beginning with a look at the history of my first medical aphorism.

Primum Non Nocere

I am sure that some aphorisms arise in their final form, like Athena spring-ing fully formed from the head of Zeus. Others, however, evolve over time. *Primum non nocere* is one of the latter. Over the years, this aphorism's significance has become more meaningful to me as I have had more and more opportunities to make occasionally harmful errors. I am well aware that I am not alone, and medicine today has taken a keen interest in medical errors, which sometimes yield profoundly harmful results. Some medical mistakes, as in the celebrated 1984 Libby Zion case in a New York hospital, can be attributed to overwork and sleep deprivation. In far too many cases, errors of omission occur because the doctor is simply too busy. Sometimes, an injurious error occurs because the doctor lacks a key bit of information, fails to make a timely referral, or sees the patient just a little too early or too late in the disease.

The "First, do no harm" admonition reminds me of a favorite quotation of L.J. Henderson (1878–1942): "Somewhere between 1910 and 1912 in this country, a random patient, with a random disease, consulting a doctor chosen at random had, for the first time in the history of mankind, a better than fifty-fifty chance of profiting from the encounter" (Strauss, p. 302). In fact, the key medical innovation of that era seems to have been the 1910 introduction of arsphenamine, an arsenic derivative marketed under the name Salvarsan for the treatment of syphilis; I don't believe that this drug tipped the clinical encounter benefit in the patient's favor very much at all. There was, in fact, a noteworthy decline in morbidity and mortality in the first half of the 20th century. Between 1900 and 1930, the average life expec-tancy of a person born in the U.S. increased from 49 to 59 years. However, these advances can be attributed chiefly to public health measures—better sanitation, improved diet, and so forth. The individual doctor, whether chosen at random or even after careful fact-finding, had little to do with the improved life expectancy. The days of breathtaking pharmacologic and technical marvels were yet to come. I would put the tipping point at about three decades later, when effective antibiotics came into use. But you get the point. As I will point out in chapter 11, we have taken many wrong turns on the way to today's evidence-based clinical care.

But let us return to our aphorism about avoiding harm. According to Smith, the "so-called Hippocratic injunction to do no harm has been an axiom central to clinical pharmacology and to the education of medical and graduate students" (5). You will find that the phrase is often attributed to Hippocrates. In fact, Hippocrates' *Epidemics* (Book I, section XI) states, "As to diseases, make a habit of two things—to help, or at least to do no harm" (Strauss, p. 625). The Hippocratic Oath—recently the victim of a great deal of linguistic revisionism—directs the physician to "abstain from whatever is deleterious or mischievous." Thus, Hippocrates certainly embraced the "Above all, do no harm" aphorism, even if the precise lan-guage may be lacking in his writings.

There is, however, an earlier source. In the Oath of the Hindu Physician (ca. 1500 BCE), we find the admonition, ". . . do the sick no harm . . ." (Strauss, p. 325). This oath predates Hippocrates by some 1,000 years or more.

Others believe that in the second century Galen (129–200) played a role in shaping the aphorism. Also, in Smith's scholarly article, he reports "the appearance of the axiom as expressed in English, coupled with its unique Latin, in 1860, with attribution to the English physician, Thomas Sydenham" (5). Florence Nightingale (1820–1910) remarked that the very first requirement of a hospital is that it should do the sick no harm. Yes, for centuries, even millennia, healers have shared this admonition with generations of aspiring physicians, leading eventually to the surgeon who wrote "*Primum non nocere*" on the blackboard in my classroom in 1957. Then, in 1992, in the television show *Northern Exposure*, the young rural physician-hero told America that, "Whatever we diagnose, most patients, if they don't die, get well by themselves. Our job is mainly to make them feel better; do no harm." The phrase has taken a long journey over the past 3,500 years.

Three Timeless Aphorists

If you search the Web for medical aphorisms, three names stand out among the responses. These are Hippocrates, Maimonides, and Osler.

The Aphorisms of Hippocrates

Hippocrates (ca. 460–377 BCE), described by legend as a direct descendent of Aesculapius, the ancient Greek god of medicine, may be considered the father of the medical aphorism. His book *Aphorisms* contains interpretations of health and disease and the relationship of both to nature. Considering the belief systems of the time, and the paucity of technology and formal research, the observations in the book are often astounding. Here are a few examples of the insights of Hippocrates (2):

- "Persons who are naturally very fat are apt to die earlier than those who are slender." Remember that Hippocrates made this observation two millennia before the concept of the heart attack was elucidated. For many subsequent years in history, people believed that there was some sort of virtue in corpulence. Being what we would consider overweight signified that one had the resources to obtain and consume more food than body needs required.

  As I thought about this aphorism, I considered some legendary obese persons. Henry VIII of England (1491–1547) was grossly overweight when he died of heart failure at age 55. William Howard Taft (1857–1930), weighing more than 350 pounds, was America's heaviest president. More recently, actor John Candy (1950–1994), who weighed more than 300 pounds, died suddenly of a heart attack while making a film in Durango, Mexico. Candy was 44 years old when he died.

- "In every movement of the body, whenever one begins to endure pain, it will be relieved by rest." Today, rest is the first element of the RICE (Rest, Ice, Compression, Elevation) acronym for treating acute musculoskeletal injuries.
- "Persons who have had frequent and severe attacks of swooning, without any manifest cause, die suddenly." Of course, the 21st century doctor, when faced with a patient with recurrent fainting, will think of cardiac arrhythmia, hypotension, transient ischemic attacks, anemia, uncontrolled diabetes, and more. Hippocrates, with little knowledge of these specific diseases and with only his powers of observation, correctly noted the risks attendant to repeated episodes of unconsciousness.
- "Old persons have fewer complaints than the young, but those chronic diseases which do befall them generally never leave them." As I age and experience an increasing number of personal adventures into patient-hood, I note that my personal medical "problem list" just seems to grow. For the older individual, seldom is a disease removed from the list; it is merely modified with the descriptor "chronic."
- "It is better that a fever succeed to a convulsion, than a convulsion to fever." Perhaps many of the former were undoubtedly febrile convulsions—certainly an alarming event but usually without dire consequences. A convulsion followed by a fever, however, conjures up images of a brain abscess, a stroke complicated by pneumonia, or a severe infectious disease with the convulsion as an early manifestation.
- "In acute diseases it is not quite safe to prognosticate either death or recovery." Amen! In more recent times, this admonition was restated by Albert R. Lamb: "Patients and their families will forgive you for wrong prognoses; the older you grow in medicine, the more chary you get about offering iron-clad prognoses, good or bad" (Strauss, p. 461).

The six sayings discussed above are only a small sample; Table 7.1 lists some other aphorisms of Hippocrates (2,3).

TABLE 7.1. Other Aphorisms Attributed to Hippocrates

When sleep puts an end to delirium, it is a good sign.
Both sleep and insomnolency, when immoderate, are bad.
Spontaneous lassitude indicates disease.
Those bodies which have been slowly emaciated should be slowly recruited; and those that have been quickly emaciated should be quickly recruited.
What remains in diseases after the crisis is apt to produce relapses.
When in a state of hunger, one ought not to undertake labor.
Acute diseases come to a crisis in fourteen days.
Drinking strong wine cures hunger.
A woman does not take the gout, unless her menses be stopped.
Pains and fevers occur rather at the formation of pus than when it is already formed.
Of two pains occurring together, not in the same part of the body, the stronger weakens the other.

The Aphorisms of Moses Maimonides

Moses Maimonides was born in Spain in 1135, spent some of his adult years in Jerusalem, and eventually settled in Cairo, where he was physician to the Sultan Saladin of Egypt. He became the spiritual leader of the Egyptian Jewish community, and in 1178, he penned a 14-volume compilation encompassing Talmudic and biblical law (6).

Maimonides' contribution to medicine included 10 medical works, as described in chapter 1. Maimonides championed the concept of "a healthy mind in a healthy body" (6). *The Medical Aphorisms of Moses* is comprised of 25 treatises containing 1,500 sayings.

Aphorisms contributed to posterity by Maimonides include the following (7):

- "No disease that can be treated by diet should be treated by any other means." This aphorism has stood the test of time. Today, the current report of the Joint Committee on Detection, Evaluation and Treatment of Hypertension recommends diet and other lifestyle changes as the foundation of management, to be used whenever possible before drugs are added.
- "Teach your tongue to say 'I do not know' and you will progress." A willingness to admit a lack of information is the first step in clinical inquiry and sets the stage for formulating the all-important research question. Admitting "I don't know" also helps the physician avoid the appearance of understanding a patient's illness when in fact one does not. We have classified sarcoidosis as an autoimmune disorder; does this mean that we really understand its nature? We can name amyloidosis, but what really is the cause? Patients with Alzheimer disease, at autopsy, have neurofibrillary tangles in the brain tissue, but does knowing this fact mean we comprehend the disease? Several centuries later, Osler would echo Maimonides' saying: "I have learned since to be a better student and to be ready to say to my fellow students 'I do not know.'" Today, being willing to admit uncertainty can help avoid leading patients to believe that you know more than you do and that you can deliver cures that are beyond your, or anyone's, abilities.
- "(In treating the sick), the first thing to consider is the provision of fresh air, clean water, and a healthy diet." Recall the notorious "window tax" enacted in 1696 in England, a law that imposed property taxes on homes according to the number of windows in the dwelling. In response, homes soon came to have few windows, inviting stale air and dampness. Garrison states, "This tyrannous tax on light and air (abolished 1851) was an activator of infection in dark houses throughout the 18th century" (8).
- "With an illness affecting the lungs, ... namely phthisis, there develops rounding of the nail as a rainbow." Today, we describe the nail rounding as clubbing or hypertrophic pulmonary osteoarthropathy.

TABLE 7.2. Other Aphorisms of Moses Maimonides

It is impossible for the strength of an elderly person to be great. Some physicians think that
   children also do not have great strength, but they are mistaken in their opinion.
The nose is the first and foremost instrument of respiration.
Twitching occurs in all parts that can stretch, but never occurs in bones and cartilages,
   because bones and cartilages do not stretch in any way.
The penis, genitalia, and neck of the uterus are reached by a surplus of nerves because of
   the extra sensation which they need during sexual intercourse.
The strongest cause in the generation of diseases is the predisposition of the body which is
   likely to fall ill.
It is in all cases unavoidable that the heart is afflicted when death occurs.
Inequality of the pulse is in most cases accompanied by irregularity; one hardly ever finds a
   regular unequal pulse.
Any urine that turns black is so extremely malignant that I do not know anyone who has
   micturated black urine and survived.

- "The basic symptoms which occur in pneumonia and which are never
  lacking are acute fever, sticking pain in the side, short rapid breaths, ser-
  rated pulse, and cough, mostly with sputum." Not much has changed in
  2,500 years.
- "The worst city is that which is sheltered from the east winds and in which
  hot and cold winds blow." Could Maimonides have been discussing air
  pollution? Certainly, Los Angeles and a few other cities in California
  could benefit from some east winds—whether hot or cold—to clear out
  the smog.

Table 7.2 lists other clinical observations of Maimonides (6,7,9).

When Maimonides died in December 1204, Jews, Christians, and Muslims
alike mourned him. According to legend, his body was placed on a donkey,
which was set free to wander. Eventually, the donkey stopped in Tiberius,
a city along the 32-mile shoreline of the Sea of Galilee, and Maimonides
was buried there (6).

The Aphorisms of Sir William Osler

Sir William Osler (1849–1919), Canadian physician, medical historian, and
teacher, is described in the *Columbia Encyclopedia* as the most brilliant and
influential teacher of medicine of his day. I consider Osler to be one of
medicine's heroes, and his exploits are described in chapter 1. Here, I want
to discuss Osler's contributions to medicine's collections of aphorisms.

Osler raised the aphorism to an art form, using wit, irony, and metaphor.
Consider the imagery in this saying: "To study the phenomenon of disease
without books is to sail uncharted sea, while to study books without patients
is not to go to sea at all." Many of Osler's sayings were collected by Robert
Bennett Bean, MD (1874–1944) and edited by William Bennett Bean, MD
(10). The following are some "Oslerisms" that influence medicine even
today:

- "It is much more important to know what sort of patient has a disease than what sort of disease the patient has." Consider that this saying anticipated the (w)holistic medicine movement by at least half a century. And Osler was an internist whose published works included observation of the elevated red blood cell count in polycythemia. Of course, Osler lived and wrote in the days when, as mentioned above, a random patient, with a random disease, consulting a doctor chosen at random was placing his health at risk. Today, when we have breathtaking medical technology and astoundingly potent medications, the best clinical outcomes still occur when the physician understands both disease and patient.
- "The desire to take medicine is perhaps the greatest feature which distinguishes man from animals." Osler espoused therapeutic parsimony, or at least prudence, and in his teaching often returned to the theme of avoiding overmedication. Two such examples are "One of the first duties of the physician is to educate the masses not to take medicine," and more colorfully, "Nickel-in-the slot, press-the-button therapeutics are no good. You cannot have a drug for every malady" (Strauss, p. 125).

In his thoughts about therapeutics, Osler was ahead of his time for three reasons. One is that medication is always a two-edged sword—capable of both helping and harming. Any drug with the power to heal can have significant side effects that may reveal themselves only over time. Witness the withdrawal of the cyclooxygenase-2 (COX-2) inhibitor rofecoxib (Vioxx) after widespread use revealed the risk of cardiovascular disease. We will return to therapeutic misadventures in chapter 11.

Second, sometimes our drugs become less useful when used excessively. Osler quipped, "One should treat as many patients as possible with a new drug while it still has the power to heal." I suspect that he was alluding to the enthusiasm that inevitably accompanies the release of a new drug. Had he lived a century later, he might have been discussing the overuse of antibiotic agents. For years, we believed that we could continue to discover new, more powerful antibiotics faster than the microorganisms could develop resistance. Today, we have learned better and we are paying the price for past folly, as the common bacterial causes of cystitis and acute exacerbations of chronic bronchitis have evolved to exhibit a worrisome resistance to the various antimicrobials we have depended upon for years.

I think Osler was also keenly aware that the healing power of the physician in the sickroom could often trump the most potent medication. Whether the patient received a tablet, an injection, or simply reassurance, the physician's presence has profound therapeutic properties. In his book *The Doctor, His Patient and the Illness*, Balint presents the insightful concept that often the doctor is the drug. He goes on to write that, "The drug 'doctor' is evidently far from being standardized. What is still more interesting is that patients can benefit from all these varieties of the drug" (11). Yes, the doctor at the bedside can often accomplish what the latest, highly promoted antimicrobial or chemotherapeutic agent cannot.

- "Superfluity of lecturing causes ischial bursitis." In case this aphorism is not clear to all, here is another on the topic of lectures and lecturing: "The dissociation of student and patient is a legacy of the pernicious system of theoretical teaching." Osler was a gifted medical educator with a strong commitment to clinically grounded teaching based on sound scientific principles. In his attention to scientific principles, he exemplified what Flexner espoused in 1910 (see chapter 1). But Osler's particular emphasis was the approach to the patient: "In what may be called the natural method of teaching, the student begins with the patient, continues with the patient, and ends with the patient, using books and lectures as tools, a means to an end."

  Over the past decade, progressive medical schools have undergone predictably painful curriculum revisions intended to reduce didactic teaching in favor of patient-centered experiential education. These schools took to heart Osler's advice to students: "Do not waste the hours of daylight in listening to that which you may read by night." Our medical school in Oregon undertook this huge change about 15 years ago, experiencing the true meaning of the educational aphorism: "Changing a medical school curriculum is like moving a graveyard." But we succeeded, and our students no longer—as I did in the 1950s—spend 8-hour days in dark lecture halls developing ischial bursitis. Osler would be proud.

- "A physician who treats himself has a fool for a patient." (And a version I have heard adds ". . . and a fool for a doctor.") I include this Oslerism here, first, to credit Sir William as the original author of this oft-quoted saying. I have searched and can find no earlier source. Second, is this admonition as precisely true today as it was a century ago? Today, with ready access to medical information over the Internet, physicians as well as lay patients can study their diseases in depth and become knowledgeable partners in health care decisions. And so, while global treatment strategies should certainly involve appropriate physician consultation, most physicians make some day-by-day tactical decisions for themselves and their families.

- "Common sense in medical matters is rare and is usually in inverse ratio to the degree of education." The best doctor is generally the one who pays attention to the patient, follows up test results carefully, and looks up the details of recommended therapy. Sometimes these doctors perform poorly on multiple-choice examinations, but when I am sick, I would prefer the common-sense physician to one who performs brilliantly on standardized tests.

- "No more dangerous members of our profession exist than those born into it, so to speak, as specialists." Osler's aphorism seems to agree with the definition of Dr. William J. Mayo: "Specialist: a man who knows more and more about less and less." Osler was very concerned about the tendency—even in his day—for young physicians to specialize too early in their careers. He believed that, "The incessant concentration of thought

TABLE 7.3. Other Aphorisms of Sir William Osler

The good observer is not limited to the large hospital.

As no two faces, so no two cases are alike in all respects, and unfortunately it is not only the disease itself which is so varied, but the subjects themselves have peculiarities which modify its action.

Soap and water and common sense are the best disinfectants.

Jaundice is the disease that your friends diagnose.

What can one hear with one's fingers? Vocal fremitus and a sharp second sound.

A great university has a dual function, to teach and to think.

Always look at the feet. Looking at a woman's legs has often saved her life.

No bubble is so iridescent or floats longer than that blown by the successful teacher.

It is a common error to think that the more a doctor sees the greater his experience and the more he knows.

There are only two sorts of doctors, those that practice with their brains, and those who practice with their tongues.

We are constantly misled by the ease with which our minds fall into the ruts of one or two experiences.

If the license to practice meant the completion of education, how sad it would be for the young practitioner, how distressing for his patients!

upon one subject, however interesting, tethers a man's mind in a narrow field." He was an advocate for generalism and advised students, "Have no higher ambition than to become an all-around family doctor, whose business in life is to know disease and to know how to treat it."

Table 7.3 lists some other Oslerisms (10).

Other Clinical Aphorisms

Let us move into the 21st century with some selected aphorisms that have clinical relevance today. What follows are, for the most part, sayings that have become part of the lore of medicine. The origins of some are obscure. For all, I have checked reference books and the Internet to try to find the original authors, but in many instances, their identities are lost in the mists of history. For this reason, my notes will sometimes tell you where I encountered them first. If any readers can clarify the original sources of the aphorisms presented without attribution, I would be grateful.

About Diagnosis

"When you hear hoofbeats, look for horses, not zebras."

In other words, the most common things occur most commonly. The often-cited zebra aphorism has been attributed to Dr. Theodore E. Woodward (1914–2005) of the University of Maryland (12). As the tale goes, Dr.

Woodward cautioned medical students and residents in the 1940s, "Don't look for zebras on Greene Street." Greene Street in Baltimore is the address of the University of Maryland Hospital.

The zebra aphorism is—in a sense—a medical restatement of Occam's razor. William of Occam was a 14th century English logician and Franciscan friar. His principle, sometimes called the law of economy, is roughly translated from Latin as, "Of two equivalent theories or explanations, all other things being equal, the simpler one is to be preferred." A century later, Leonardo da Vinci observed, "Simplicity is the ultimate sophistication." Today, our young people use the KISS principle—Keep It Simple, Stupid. As a clinical corollary, experienced diagnosticians look first for uncommon manifestations of common conditions rather than common manifestations of uncommon diseases. Whatever your favorite iteration of the simplicity theorem, keeping horses and zebras in mind will help you avoid overlooking the most likely diagnoses.

"Listen to the patient; he or she is telling you the diagnosis."

If there is a secret to making the correct diagnosis, it is allowing patients to tell their stories, in their own words, with all the verbal inflections, facial expressions, and body language. We physicians, living our professional lives under (often self-induced) time pressures, move too quickly to focused "yes-no" questions and often fail to experience the nuances of the patient's narrative. Furthermore, in our new age of magnetic resonance imaging and positron emission tomography, it is easy to forget the value of a good medical history.

"All that wheezes is not asthma."

This is attributed to Chevalier Jackson, MD (1865–1958), renowned pulmonologist at Temple University School of Medicine, whom my professors considered the father of bronchoscopy. Jackson is also the source of the maxim that "In teaching the medical student, the primary requisite is to keep him awake." I attended Temple University School of Medicine, but sufficiently long after the days of Dr. Jackson that his "keeping the student awake" observation could not have been in reference to me.

"Adhesions are the refuge of the diagnostically destitute."

Over the years, this quip by Sir William Osler has helped me and my residents revise our differential diagnoses for some patients with recurrent abdominal pain.

"The doctor who makes the correct diagnosis will be the one who sees the patient last."

Patients and physicians alike often fail to recall that disease evolves and serious, chronic diseases almost always progress. Hence, the manifestations

of, for example, breast cancer or coronary artery disease which are quite apparent today may not have been detectable when the patient was examined by another doctor at some point in the past. When you think about it, it is usually the subspecialist who gets to see the patient last, often after a valiant attempt at diagnosis by the generalist, who eventually seeks subspecialist consultation.

"A smart mother often makes a better diagnosis than a poor doctor."

This is attributed to August Bier (1861–1949). Parents are often right on target with their diagnostic impressions. Access to medical information on the Internet is making experts of us all. Certainly, the astute physician will want to learn the mother's (or father's) diagnostic impression, if only to include it among the possibilities that are excluded on the way to the correct conclusion. And remember: sometimes Mom will be right.

"The fact that the patient gets well does not prove that your diagnosis was correct."

God and Mother Nature will cure most ailments, regardless of whether we have applied the correct Latin name or our favorite remedy.

About Treatment

"It is difficult to make the asymptomatic patient feel better."

This aphorism is from an article by Hoerr (13), cited in Strauss (p. 638). When treating the "worried well person," it is especially important to remember that all interventions have consequences, even lifestyle changes. I always think of this aphorism when I initiate drug therapy for hypertension. Most hypertensive patients feel just fine, thank you. We are asking them to take daily medication on the assurance that they will lessen their statistical risk of a stroke or some other complication in the future. The anti-hypertensive drugs, however, can cause fatigue, nocturia, dizziness, or even sexual dysfunction. Now the patient, although perhaps normotensive, is no longer asymptomatic. Now he or she has some symptoms—correction, side effects—that interfere with the quality of life.

"Treat the patient, not the x-ray."

This is a favorite aphorism of orthopedic surgeons and others who treat patients with fractures. Another helpful saying regarding fracture management is, "A wiggle a day keeps the callus away." If you want a broken bone to heal firmly, be sure that the fragments are correctly aligned and then held in this position by stable immobilization.

"In a patient age 90 or above, all findings on a chest film taken with the patient standing are considered normal."

This wry observation somehow seems reasonable. On the other hand, I cannot agree with a radiologist's alleged comparison of the x-ray with the stethoscope: "One look is worth a thousand listens."

"It takes two years to learn when to enter the abdominal cavity and 20 years to learn when to stay out."

Surgery is a pet topic of clinical aphorisms. Robert L. Tait (1845–1899) wrote, "When in doubt, drain." And from William S. Halsted (1852–1922) comes, "The only weapon with which the unconscious patient can immediately retaliate upon the incompetent surgeon is hemorrhage." And finally, when considering whether a procedure is needed, "The lesser the indication, the greater the complication."

"If your only tool is a hammer, everything you see looks like a nail."

If your patient's coronary artery disease could be treated equally well with medication or with surgery, the therapeutic path may well be determined by which specialist you consult. Medical specialists medicate; surgeons operate.

Timeless Clinical Aphorisms

"Children are not simply micro-adults, but have their own specific problems."

Bela Schick (1877–1967), who devised a skin test for susceptibility to *Corynebacterium diphtheriae*, coined this saying. Dr. Schick might have added that children can have special peculiarities when it comes to drug doses.

"Rheumatic fever licks at the joint, but bites at the heart."

This saying is attributed to Ernest C. Lasègue (1816–1883), who devised the Lasègue sign for sciatic nerve root irritation. Recall the five major Jones criteria for the diagnosis of rheumatic fever: polyarthritis, carditis, chorea, erythema marginatum, and subcutaneous nodules. The "arthritis" of rheumatic fever will subside, but the carditis may cause lifelong problems.

"Varicose veins are the result of an improper selection of grandparents."

This is attributed to Sir William Osler. Osler might have added a few other hereditary maladies, such as diabetes mellitus, coronary artery disease, genetic short stature, and flat feet.

"Pneumonia is the old man's friend."

For centuries, pneumonia allowed the aged and feeble a gentle exit at the end of life. Today, we have the Pneumovax paradox. By administering pneumococcal vaccine to infirm elderly persons (including many with dementia in nursing homes), we deny them the "old man's friend."

Other Selected Medical Aphorisms

In this chapter, we have seen how the medical aphorism has evolved from an insightful generalization, often one that summarized many individual clinical observations into a memorable and sometimes clever statement of a general truth. Over the years, the neoaphorisms that endured were often droll, ironic, or even sardonic. Here, in the last section of the chapter, I will present some aphorisms that exhibit these characteristics.

About Doctoring

"Good judgment comes from experience; experience comes from bad judgment."

This is attributed to Kerr L. White (1917–). Yes, the physician who makes poor decisions is likely to experience more disease and surgical complications than one who makes good decisions. We hope that good judgment would follow; alas, such is not always the case. Another viewpoint is, "Experience is what you rely on when you haven't read anything for a while" (14).

"The patient in front of you in the exam room is not the average patient from whom statistics were compiled."

This aphorism is cited by Reveno (p. 105).

"The physician as a patient will get every possible complication."

We are all well aware not only that this aphorism is true, but that it extends to all members of the physician's family. Doctors are also destined to get the rare and wonderful diseases: "A rare disease is something you will never diagnose yourself, but if you live long enough, you will probably get one" (14).

But it seems that we can worry a little less about physicians' family members. "No member of a physician's family ever had an illness that could not be adequately treated with something in the drug sample cabinet."

"There are some patients whom we cannot help; there are none whom we cannot harm."

The author of this saying, writing in the 1930s following a medical error, held that every hospital should have a plaque containing these words at the entrance for students and physicians (A.L. Bloomfield, cited in Strauss, p. 636).

Academic Medicine Aphorisms

Academic medicine is a special room in the house of medicine. Here we find a society of physicians and others which has its own culture, traditions, and rules of engagement. For the community-based physician, the academic medical center (AMC)—medical school and the teaching hospital—was a stopping point on the journey into actual practice. For those who spend their careers in teaching and research, the AMC is their reality. In an effort to tell my vision of this reality, I wrote a book entitled *Academic Medicine: A Guide for Clinicians*, and in this book, I discussed some of the aphorisms popular with academic clinicians (15). Here are a few of them:

"If you have seen one academic medical center, you have seen one."

Although AMCs all share some activities—teaching, doing research, and providing patient care—each is unique in special ways. Examples include the Byzantine organizational hierarchy, the relationship of the medical school and teaching hospital, the governance of the faculty practice, and the ways in which faculty are promoted and tenured.

"The three priorities in teaching are first, to inspire; second, to challenge; and third and only third, to impart information."

This aphorism is cited by Bishop (16). Young teachers want to tell everything they know. Mature educators recognize the value of motivated self-learning.

"To teach is to learn twice."

This aphorism is attributed to Joseph Joubert (1754–1824), French moralist and essayist. Anyone who has ever prepared a lecture to present to a classroom of students or taught a resident in the office understands this truism. Furthermore, some days I think I learn more from my students than I teach them. For those who like aphorisms, here is another by Joubert: "When you go in search of honey, you must expect to be stung by bees."

"When you're talking, you aren't learning anything."

This aphorism is attributed to U.S. President Lyndon B. Johnson (1908–1973). Many medical educators (and, for that matter, many physicians) talk when they should be listening. The most skillful communicators listen much more than they talk. And those speaking with these individuals think they are brilliant. Just for listening.

"Good writing can't fix poor research."

The final step of a research project is to have the findings published in a prestigious medical journal, which calls for a meticulously written article that will be scrutinized by peer reviewers. But this is not where research goes wrong. Problems are most likely to arise far upstream as the project is conceptualized. Early missteps, such a poor study design or biased sample selection, cannot be corrected later in writing up the findings.

On a slightly cynical note about research: "Clinicians ask the right questions incorrectly; researchers ask the wrong questions, but do so correctly." Or as someone once said, "It is fine in practice, but it will never work in theory."

And just for fun: "A university is a loose confederation of departments united by a common parking problem." A friend from Florida told me that in that state, the unifying link is the air-conditioning ducts.

Some Humorous Aphorisms

Some medical aphorisms cross over the line from witty to downright funny. Here are a few I have heard over the years. Most are from unknown origins.

"In an emergency, first take your own pulse."
"Bleeding always stops." Sooner or later, the surgeon will ligate a bleeder, the clotting mechanism will stop the flow of blood, or the patient will exsanguinate.
"Cancer cures smoking."
"Never trust a naked baby." No experienced clinician (or parent) would stand "downstream" from an undiapered male infant.
"A two-year-old is a psychopathic dwarf with a good prognosis." And later in life: "An adolescent is a schizophrenic with a good prognosis" (Thomas L. Coleman, cited in Brallier, p. 42).
"Insanity is hereditary; we get it from our children."
"The number of tubes in a patient is inversely related to the prognosis."
"Every hypochondriacal patient eventually dies of a physical disease."

For some truly irreverent and cutting aphorisms, read Shem's novel *The House of God* (17). Several of Shem's aphorisms concern the GOMER, an acronym for "Get Out of My Emergency Room" (see chapter 6). Here are House of God "rules" that have become part of today's hospital culture:

- "GOMERs don't die."
- "GOMERs go to ground." That is, they tend to fall out of bed or off the edge of gurneys.

- "Placement comes first." At the moment a patient is admitted, you should begin discharge planning.
- "The delivery of medical care is to do as much nothing as possible." Could this be a restatement of "First, do no harm"?

To end this chapter, here is an aphorism that appears on a plaque high on the wall in our conference room: "Asking stupid questions is much better than correcting dumb mistakes." *Primum non nocere.*

References

1. Fabing H, Marr R. *Fischerisms*. Springfield, IL: Charles C. Thomas; 1944.
2. Hippocrates. *Aphorisms*. Available at: http://classics.mit.edu/Hippocrates/aphorisms.html. Accessed May 16, 2007.
3. Hippocrates. *The Aphorisms of Hippocrates*. Cambridge, MA: DevCom; 1987.
4. Geary J. *The World in a Phrase: A Brief History of the Aphorism*. London, UK: Bloomsbury Publishing; 2005.
5. Smith CM. Origin and uses of primum non nocere–above all, do no harm! *J Clin Pharmacol*. 2005;45;371–377.
6. Rosner F. The life of Moses Maimonides, a prominent medieval physician. *Einstein Q J Biol Med*. 2002;19:125–128.
7. Rosner F, Muntner S. *The Medical Aphorisms of Moses Maimonides*. New York, NY: Yeshiva University; 1970.
8. Garrison FH. *History of Medicine*. 4th ed. Philadelphia, PA: Saunders; 1929.
9. Maimonides. *Medical Aphorisms: Treatises 1–5*. Bos G, trans. Provo, UT: Brigham Young University Press; 2004.
10. Bean RB, Bean WB. *Sir William Osler: Aphorisms from his bedside teachings and writings*. Springfield, IL: Charles C. Thomas; 1961.
11. Balint M. *The Doctor, His Patient and the Illness*. Millennium edition. London, UK: Churchill Livingstone; 2000:5.
12. Who coined the aphorism? Available at: http://www.zebracards.com/a-intro_inventor.html. Accessed May 14, 2007.
13. Hoerr SO. Hoerr's law. *Am J Surg*. 1962;103:411.
14. Bennett HJ. Humor in the medical literature. *J Fam Pract*. 1995;40:334–336.
15. Taylor RB. *Academic Medicine: A Guide for Clinicians*. New York, NY: Springer Verlag Publishers; 2006.
16. Bishop JM. Infuriating tensions: science and the medical student. *J Med Educ*. 1984;59:91–102.
17. Shem S. *The House of God*. New York, NY: Dell; 1981.

8
Memorable Medical Quotations

Winston Churchill once wrote, "It is a good thing for an uneducated man to read books of quotations." I believe that it is perhaps even better for presumably educated persons, such as physicians, to read insightful quotations said and written by our predecessors. These quotes are a valuable part of our heritage, and they afford insights into the thinking of yesterday's great men and women of medicine. If nothing else, they will expand your consciousness, enhance your vocabulary, and help you become a more thoughtful physician.

As you look for meaningful medical quotations, which I earnestly hope you will do, you will find the medical landscape full of them. Through the years, physicians and scientists have uttered many quotable thoughts, and, being learned individuals, have often done so in quite articulate ways. If you search the literature for medical sayings, you soon discover what I believe is the classic reference book: *Familiar Medical Quotations* by Strauss (the full citation is in the Bibliography list). Strauss' book contains more than 7,000 quotations, including six by the compiler himself. Many of the quotations in this chapter can be found in Strauss' book.

What makes a memorable medical quote? Amidst all the pedantic drivel found in the thousands of medical articles that litter the publication landscape each year, there are a few—and only a very few—insightful gems of wisdom that merit recalling, inscribing in your journal, and citing in your next lecture or paper. These precious few wise words are the memorable medical quotations bound to be mentioned with attribution, collected in quotation books, and ultimately paraphrased and plagiarized. These quotations will transcend the articles in which they originally occur and in the end will outlive their authors. What makes such a saying?

After reviewing hundreds of medical quotations in organizing this chapter, I conclude that our best medical quotations have the following attributes:

- Originality. A memorable quotation must be not only the author's words, but also his or her idea. For example, generations of medical authors have probably exhausted the ways to say, "First, do no harm" and "Chance favors only the prepared mind."

- Succinctness. The most enduring quotations are not too long. To be remembered and subsequently quoted, a saying must be of reasonable length. The highly complex sentence, chock full of commas and subordinate clauses, may precisely express a brilliant thought, but the words are likely to be difficult to recall. Brevity trumps verbosity.
- Simplicity. Great quotations are easy to comprehend. They generally use short, easy-to-understand words. As Churchill once said, "Short words are best, and the old words when short are best of all."
- Imagery. "Words are for people that can't read pictures," said Pogo, title character in the comic strip by Walt Kelly. But words can paint pictures in the mind. Here is a good example of a visual image, this one in a quotation attributed to Raymond Whitehead (1904–1965): "Medicine is not a field in which sheep may safely graze" (Strauss, p. 304).
- Universality. If a quotation is to be meaningful in varied cultures and to endure from one generation to the next, it must convey some sort of universal truth. A brilliant saying about a time-limited phenomenon—such as a health care proposal before Congress or today's therapy of AIDS—is unlikely to be recalled a decade from now.

With thousands of medical quotations to choose from, how should I approach this chapter? My goal, as in the other chapters in the book, is to give the reader a sampling of the wealth of available material—whether quotations, aphorisms, acronyms, or historical anecdotes. Still, the biopsy material must be organized somehow. To put some structure to my selection of noteworthy medical quotations, I have elected to present sayings that fall into one of three areas: some quotations from the historical heroes described in chapter 1; an assortment of thoughts worth remembering about medicine, life, death, and doctors; and I will end the chapter, as dessert, with a few humorous quotations about medicine as a profession.

Quotations Attributed to Some of Medicine's Heroes

The quotations in this section span 2,500 years. In one manner or another, all have to do with medicine. I present these to offer insight into the minds of our heroes in an effort to add context to their accomplishments.

What Our Heroes Said

Greco-Roman Medicine

In the fifth century BCE, Hippocrates (ca. 460–377 BCE) spoke of the relationship of persons, disease, and nature. "Natural forces are the healers of disease." Also attributed to him is the saying, "The art [of medicine] has three factors, the disease, the patient and the physician. The physician is the servant of the art. The patient must cooperate with the physician in combating the disease." And, "Wherever the art of medicine is loved, there is also the love of humanity."

Half a millennium later, Claudius Galen (120–200 CE), who worked to systematize medicine in his day, made this observation: "Those things which bring about health where it does not exist are called medicines and remedies, while those which maintain it where it exists are called healthy modes of living." On a more down-to-earth note, he tells us, "Confidence and hope do more good than physic."

The Middle Ages

Rhazes (850–923), both philosopher and observer, wrote, "Truth in medicine is an attainable goal, and the art as described in books is far beneath the knowledge of an experienced and thoughtful physician." Rhazes also gave us an insight that surely holds true today: "The patient who consults a great many physicians is likely to have a very confused state of mind."

Avicenna (980–1037) stated, "An ignorant doctor is the aide-de-camp of death."

Almost three centuries later, Moses Maimonides (1135–1204) said, "Medical practice is not knitting and weaving and the labor of the hands, but it must be inspired with soul and be filled with understanding and equipped with the gift of keen observation; these together with accurate scientific knowledge are the indispensable requisites for proficient medical practice."

Renaissance and Reformation in the 15th and 16th Centuries

As the Western world awoke from its medieval slumber, we begin to find some more "scientific" quotations. A transitional figure was Paracelsus (1493–1542), who postulated a "life force" ruled by nature. Paracelsus said, "The physician is only the servant of nature, not her master. Therefore, it behooves medicine to follow the will of nature."

Ambroise Paré (1517–1590), who revolutionized battlefield surgery, wrote, "Five things are proper to the duty of a Chirurgeon: to take away that which is superfluous; to restore to their places such things as are displaced; to separate those things which are joined together; to join those that are separated; and to supply the defects of nature." On a more philosophical theme, he believed that the doctor should, "Always give the patient hope, even when death seems at hand."

Paré's contemporary was Vesalius (1514–1564), the anatomist at the medical school at Padua who dissected human bodies and refuted Galenic misconceptions that had endured from Greco-Roman times to the Middle Ages. Vesalius wrote in his book *De Humanis Corporis Fabrica*, "How much has been attributed to Galen, easily leader of the professors of dissection, by those physicians and anatomists who have followed him, and often against reason. . . . there is that blessed and wonderful *plexus reticularis* which man everywhere inculcates in his books. There is nothing of which physicians speak more often. They have never seen it (for it is almost non-existent in the human body), yet they describe it from Galen's teaching. Indeed, I myself cannot wonder enough at my own stupidity and too great trust in the writing of Galen and other anatomists." It is a relief to know that today we no longer see misinformation passed from one textbook to the next.

The Seventeenth Century

This century brought some of the great works of literature, art, theater, and scientific medicine. William Harvey (1578–1657) is remembered for his description of the circulation of the blood, and yet he expressed concern about how his work would be received: "What remains to be said upon the quantity and source of the blood which thus passes, is of so novel and unheard-of a character that I not only fear injury to myself from the envy of a few, but I tremble lest I have mankind at large for my enemies, so much doth wont and custom, that become as a second nature, and doctrine once sown and that hath struck deeproot, and respect for antiquity influence all men: Still the die is cast, and my trust is in my love of truth, and the candour that inheres in cultivated minds" (Strauss, p. 58).

Shortly thereafter, Thomas Sydenham (1624–1689) gave the world thoughtful descriptions of many diseases, including the eponymic Sydenham chorea. He built bridges between science and the sickroom, exemplified in his saying, "The art of medicine was to be properly learned only from its practice and exercise." Another of his memorable quotes is, "It is my nature to think where others read."

The Eighteenth Century

James Lind (1716–1794), who showed that a diet of citrus fruits and fresh vegetables could prevent scurvy, wrote, "No physician conversant with this disease at sea had undertaken to throw light on the subject." Lind did so in the best scientific method of the day.

During the 1700s, John Hunter (1728–1657) introduced science into the art of surgery, studying what happens in the body following injury and devising novel treatment methods that anticipated techniques we use today, such as in mechanical ventilation and vascular surgery. One remarkable quotation is, "This last part of surgery, namely, operations, is a reflection on the healing art; it is a tacit acknowledgment of the insufficiency of surgery. It is like an armed savage who attempts to get that by force which a civilized man would get by stratagem."

Near the end of the century, Edward Jenner (1749–1823), who advocated smallpox vaccination using cowpox, made this observation: "The deviation of man from the state in which he was originally placed by nature seems to have proved to him a prolific source of diseases." Jenner also had a wry sense of humor: "Never believe what a patient tells you his doctor has said."

The Nineteenth Century

William T.G. Morton (1819–1868), who popularized ether anesthesia following a memorable demonstration in 1846, considered himself "a man possessed of such limited talent and so many flaws." On the other hand, he had great confidence in his drug. Morton is the person who coined a word we use today when he said, "The state should, I think, be called 'anesthesia.' This signifies insensibility." Following the first operation using ether anesthesia, surgeon John C. Warren exclaimed, "Gentlemen, this is no humbug!"

The next year, Ignaz Semmelweis (1818–1865) recognized that physicians could transmit infection to women during childbirth. He wrote, "When I look back upon the past, I can only dispel the sadness which falls upon me by gazing into the happy future when the infection will be banished. . . . The conviction that such a time must inevitably sooner or later arrive will cheer my dying hour."

John Snow (1813–1858), who helped stop a cholera epidemic in London by removal of the handle of the Broad Street Pump, once said to Henry Whitehead, "You and I may not live to see the day, and my name may be forgotten when it comes, but the time will arrive when great outbreaks of cholera will be things of the past; and it is the knowledge of the way in which the disease is propagated which will cause them to disappear" (1).

In Paris, Louis Pasteur (1822–1895) worked with cholera, anthrax, and rabies—focusing his energies on prevention, rather than cures. The list of his lifetime achievements is truly remarkable. Pasteur had an explanation for his remarkable productivity: "Let me tell you the secret that has led me to my goal. My strength lies solely in my tenacity." Pasteur also had a hint of the social activism that we find prevalent in medicine today: "[I am] a man whose invincible belief is that Science and Peace will triumph over Ignorance and War, that nations will unite, not to destroy, but to build, and that the future will belong to those who will have done the most for suffering humanity." These words, spoken in 1892, are as pertinent today as they were then.

Joseph Lister (1827–1912), a pioneer in surgical antisepsis, once observed, "To intrude an unskilled hand into such a piece of Divine mechanism as the human body is indeed a fearful responsibility." He had strong words about lifelong learning for his medical students and fellow physicians: "You must always be students, learning and unlearning till your life's end, and if, gentlemen, you are not prepared to follow your profession in this spirit, I implore you to leave its ranks and betake yourself to some third-class trade."

Marie Curie, who lived and (probably) died studying "her" radium, said, "Nothing in life is to be feared; it is only to be understood," and "I am one of those who think, like Nobel, that humanity will draw more good than evil from new discoveries." Recall that Alfred Nobel (1833–1896), who instituted the Nobel Prizes, made his fortune manufacturing explosives.

Sir William Osler was a veritable font of quotations, a number of which are described as aphorisms in chapter 7. Here are a few more of his many wise sayings: "Medicine is a science of uncertainty and an art of probability." "Variability is the law of life, and as no two faces are the same, so no two bodies are alike, and no two individuals react alike and behave alike under the abnormal conditions which we know as disease." And, "The best preparation for tomorrow is to do today's work superbly well."

The Twentieth Century

The man who, in 1910, started the revolution in medical education, William Flexner (1866–1959), had this to say about the history of medicine: "From the earliest time, medicine has been a curious blend of superstition, empiricism, and that kind of sagacious observation which is the stuff out of which ultimately science is made. Of these three strands—superstition, empiricism, and observation—medicine was constituted in the days of the priest-physicians of Egypt and Babylonia; of the same three strands it is still composed. The proportions have, however, varied significantly; an increasingly alert and determined effort, running through the ages, has endeavored to expel superstition, to narrow the range of empiricism, and to enlarge, refine, and systematize the scope of observation."

Flexner then describes his goal for educational reform in medicine: "Research, untrammeled by near reference to practical ends, will go on in every properly organized medical school; its critical method will dominate all teaching whatsoever; but undergraduate instruction will be, throughout, explicitly conscious of its professional end and aim."

Alexander Fleming (1881–1955), who discovered (and almost discarded) penicillin, has this to say about the process of scientific discovery: "It is the lone worker who makes the first advance in a subject; the details may be worked out by a team, but the prime idea is due to the enterprise, thought, and perception of an individual." It is interesting to reflect that Fleming's "eureka" observation was a solo effort, but that developing the full potential of penicillin required a team. In a quotation that would have been a fitting epitaph, he once stated, "One sometimes finds what one is not looking for."

The poliomyelitis vaccine developed by Jonas Salk (1914–1995) was introduced early in my medical career. Today, most Americans have grown up taking for granted the availability of a safe and reliable immunization against the disease. In addition to leading the development of the first polio vaccine, Salk contributed some admirable quotations to our profession: "Intuition will tell the thinking mind where to look next." "There is hope in dreams, imagination, and in the courage of those who wish to make those dreams a reality." And, "I think the greatest reward for doing is the opportunity to do more."

Thoughts About Quotations

What about the selected quotations above, which begin with the Greco-Roman era and end in modern times? All were selected because they have something to do with medicine—practice, education, research, and more. Are there common threads? Can we detect recurring themes? Do we see an evolution of thought and understanding over time?

Nature

The discussion of quotations began with a quote from Hippocrates: "Natural forces are the healers of disease." Early physicians had a spiritual, almost metaphysical, view of nature. In chapter 1, we saw how this eventually spiraled into medieval hyper-religiosity, with divine causes attributed to diseases and their outcomes. In the 16th century, Paracelsus used the term "life force" and advocated that medicine "follow the will of nature." We have never been able to isolate and study "natural forces" or the "life force," but as recently as the late 20th century, Salk spoke of dreams, imagination, and courage—things physicians should never abandon in their quest for evidence-based answers. There is still much in health and healing that we cannot see, quantitate, or control with certainty. Perhaps these are today's manifestations of "natural forces."

Observation Evolves to Become Research

Hippocrates and his contemporaries were keen observers and recognized the value of critical study. They recorded the manifestations of disease, and some of their descriptions are pertinent today. Galen went so far as to experiment—notably on animals. In doing so, he went a step beyond simple observation. In the West, medical experimentation took a holiday during medieval times, but in what we now call the Middle East, Maimonides wrote of "the gift of keen observation." Then, in the 16th century, Vesalius sought anatomical truth by dissecting human bodies, searching for—among other things—the elusive "*plexus reticularis*." Sydenham told how he would "think where others read," saying (as I understand him) that he eschewed the often inaccurate texts of the time in favor of seeking new knowledge. Hunter likened the surgical operation to "an armed savage" and sought to develop a scientific basis for the art. Pasteur and the Curies experimented on humans by using vaccines and radioactive substances.

Then, in the early 20th century, Flexner called for "research, untrammeled by near reference to practical ends" in every medical school. Along the path from observation to grant-funded research publishable in peer-reviewed journals, have we lost some of the context of Hippocrates' quotation regarding the three factors in the art of medicine—the disease, the patient, and the physician?

Empiricism to Systemization to Specialization

The earliest healers relied heavily on empiricism. As we move to Greco-Roman times, we see a growing tendency to "systematize" medicine, as seen in the works of Hippocrates and Galen. After all, in those days, the scope of medical knowledge was not nearly as vast as it is today. One gifted physician could aspire to categorize it all. In the East during the Middle Ages, Rhazes and Maimonides were both prolific authors. Rhazes wrote 25 medical books; Maimonides authored 10.

By the time of the Renaissance, areas of expertise began to develop. We read about "the duty of a Chirugeon" by Paré. Vesalius was an anatomist. Today, we would probably call Sydenham a general internist and Jenner a family physician. Hunter wrote passionately about surgery. Semmelweis was an obstetrician. The last two centuries have seen the rise of career scientists such as the Curies, Fleming, and Salk, who, when he spoke of "doing more," referred to research. Osler, who wrote of "doing today's work superbly well," will surely be the last physician to single-handedly write an encyclopedic reference book covering the vast landscape of medical diseases. We have come a long way since the early shamans employed empiric disease remedies, and today we are certainly much healthier for the journey. Now if only the patient with an undifferentiated illness could have ready access to a broad-based, skilled, empathic physician.

Treatment and Prevention

The quest to prevent disease is not new. Galen advocated "healthy modes of living" to maintain health. But in early times, disease was an everyday occurrence, and physicians struggled to care for the sick and the dying, with scant time to think about prevention. Things changed in the 18th century with Lind's work on scurvy, which (by his own account) he undertook because "no physician conversant with this disease at sea had undertaken to throw light on the subject." At the end of the century, Jenner developed a reliable and safe method of vaccination. In 1854, Snow removed the fabled pump handle, helping us to understand "the way in which the disease [cholera] is propagated." In the 20th century came Salk, who believed, "Intuition will tell the thinking mind where to look next." Salk's development of the first polio vaccine must rank with Jenner's accomplishment in showing the merits of widespread immunization efforts. Prevention has achieved parity with treatment, and, in the words of Henry E. Sigerist (1891–1957), "Every child knows that prevention is not only better than cure, but also cheaper" (Strauss, p. 452).

Humility

From the beginning, physicians—at least some of them—have been both humble and aware of iatrogenesis. "Confidence and hope do more good than physic," wrote Galen. Rhazes speaks of the risks to one "who consults a great many physicians." Paracelsus reminds us, "The physician is only the servant of nature, not her master." And Paré speaks to the value of "hope," while Vesalius wonders at "my own stupidity." In the 18th century, surgeon John Hunter speaks of the "insufficiency of surgery." William T.G. Morton, who is remembered for his introduction of ether anesthesia, describes himself as having "limited talent and so many flaws." Pasteur describes his strength not in intellectual prowess, but in his "tenacity."

Allusions to Humankind

We like to think of our heroes of medicine not only as having the best minds, but also as being admirable persons. Certainly, the work of each of the medical heroes cited has, in one way or another, advanced our health. In addition, several of the quotes selected reflect a love of fellow humans. Hippocrates writes of "the love of humanity." Semmelweis dreamed of "the happy future when the infection will banished," even though he well knew that he would not live to see that day. Snow aspired to avoid outbreaks of cholera, not merely to treat one patient, but for the benefit of all. Pasteur held that "the future will belong to those who have done the most for suffering humanity," and Marie Curie thought "humanity will draw more good than evil from new discoveries."

Some Thoughts Worth Remembering: About Medicine, Life, Death, and Doctoring

The renowned men and women of medical history have left us a legacy of memorable thoughts, but many others have also contributed timeless quotations. Not all of these persons were physicians or scientists. After all, health and medical care concern all of us. Here are some quotations, selected to reflect some wise sayings about specific topics.

About the Art of Medicine

Medicine as an Art

I will begin by quoting Plato (ca. 427–347 BCE), who was born about three decades after the birth of Hippocrates. Plato wrote, "Medicine is an art, and attends to the nature and constitution of the patient, and has principles of action in each case." A few years later in Rome, Cicero (106–43 BCE) observed, "Nor do all sick persons get well, but that does not prove that there is no art of medicine."

Medicine and Experience

The art of medicine is a balance between evidence and experience. Osler was well aware of how experience (see IGBOs in chapter 6) shapes our judgment as he wrote that we are "constantly misled by the ease with which our minds fall into ruts of one or two experiences." If you, as a physician, have long prescribed antibiotics for children with acute otitis media and have been gratified to see them almost all improve on therapy, you may find it difficult to accept the conclusions of randomized clinical studies suggesting that such therapy is often unnecessary.

J. Chalmers Da Costa (1863–1933), author of the book *Modern Surgery*, once stated, "Each one of us, however old, is still an undergraduate in the school of experience. When a man thinks he has graduated, he becomes a public menace." And, "What we call experience is often a dreadful list of ghastly mistakes."

Practicing the Art of Medicine

Writing about surgery, French author Alexandre Dumas (1802–1870) offered this opinion: "A good surgeon operates with his hand, not with his heart." Advocating a more wholistic approach, American neurosurgeon Harvey Cushing (1869–1939), who described what we now call Cushing syndrome, stated, "A physician is obligated to consider more than a diseased organ, more even than the whole man—he must view the man in his world."

In England, Sir James Bryce (1838–1922), looking at medicine from the viewpoint of a politician and historian, describes medicine as "the only profession that labours incessantly to destroy the reason for its own existence." I might suggest that dentists work toward the same goal, with no more success than physicians.

British radiologist Sir Robert G. Hutchinson (1871–1960), whose name describes a malignant tumor of children, had this to say: "It is unnecessary—perhaps dangerous—in medicine to be too clever." He also admonished, "If you once get into the habit of guessing, you are diagnostically damned."

From Albert Schweitzer (1875–1965), German philosopher-physician, comes the following opinion: "It is our duty to remember at all times and anew that medicine is not only a science, but also the art of letting our own individuality interact with the individuality of the patient."

In his book *A Sceptic's Medical Dictionary*, O'Donnell writes of the role of faith in medicine as a "valuable ally in achieving a 'cure' and a dangerous enemy in assessing it" (2).

An essay that should be read by every young physician, written by Francis W. Peabody (1881–1927), appeared in the *Journal of the American Medical*

Association in 1927 (3). I will share three related thoughts from this seminal work:

"There is no more contradiction between the science of medicine and the art of medicine than between the science of aeronautics and the art of flying."

"Disease in man is never exactly the same as disease in an experimental animal, for in man the disease at once affects and is affected by what we call the emotional life. Thus, the physician who attempts to take care of a patient while he neglects this factor is as unscientific as the investigator who neglects to control all the conditions that may affect his experiment."

The concluding sentence in Peabody's article has been quoted countless times: "One of the essential qualities of the clinician is interest in humanity, for the secret of the care of the patient is in caring for the patient."

And there may be one more secret, identified by Phillips and Haynes. It is *being there* for the patient and family. In their words, "You can pretend to know, you can pretend to care, but you cannot pretend to be there." This means making time to listen to the anguished patient, showing up at the bedside even when another physician is responsible for the surgery or intensive care, and making the house call when the little voice within says that you really should (4).

About Life, Health, Disease, and Death

Very simply stated, medicine is about preventing, treating, and curing disease and enhancing health, with the goal of augmenting the quality and length of life. It is about *life*, and inevitably *death*. Some of the well-known persons in history, physicians and others, have given us insightful quotations on these topics.

Life and Health

Through the years, many of the world's great minds have addressed the topic of life. Below are some examples. Are these ideas relevant to medicine? I believe they are.

"Life is a progress, not a station." American author and philosopher Ralph Waldo Emerson (1803–1882)

"If I had to define life in a single phrase, I should clearly express my thought by throwing into relief the one characteristic which, in my opinion, sharply differentiates biological science. I would say: life is creation." French physiologist Claude Bernard (1813–1878)

"The purpose of human life is to serve and to show compassion and the will to help others." German philosopher and physician Albert Schweitzer (1875–1965)

"Life begets energy. Energy begets energy. It is by spending oneself that one becomes rich." French actress Sarah Bernhardt (1844–1923)

"Life is trying things to see if they work." American science fiction writer Ray Bradbury (born 1920)

"Let us live life so that when we die even the undertaker will be sorry." American writer Samuel Langhorne Clemens, aka Mark Twain (1835–1910)

In the end, there is dying and death, the last chapter of life. "And I looked, and behold a pale horse: and his name that sat upon him was Death" (Book of Revelation 6:8). Eventually, all our patients will die, although some will always outlive their physicians. Renaissance surgeon Ambroise Paré, faced with the recommendation that his toes be amputated, declared, "I prefer to die by the hand of God." Here are some other thoughts about death.

"A good death does honor to a whole life." Italian poet Francesco Petrarca, aka Petrarch (1304–1374)

"Worry affects the circulation, the heart, glands, the whole nervous system. I have never known a man who died from overwork, but many who died from doubt." American physician Charles H. Mayo (1865–1939)

"Dying is a very dull, dreary affair. And my advice to you is to have nothing whatsoever to do with it." British writer W. Somerset Maugham (1874–1965)

"I am ready to meet my Maker, but whether my Maker is prepared for the great ordeal of meeting me is another matter." British political leader Winston Churchill (1874–1965)

"If my doctor told me I had only six minutes to live, I wouldn't brood. I'd type a little faster." Russian-born science writer Isaac Asimov (1920–1992)

About the Doctor

Medicine, life, health, disease, and death all intersect in the encounter between the patient and the physician. It was so in the time of Hippocrates and—despite eHealth and little television-bearing robots chugging about making hospital rounds—it is so today. We, the physicians, are the persons to whom the sick and the dying look for help. Here are some thoughts about physicians.

Hippocrates is reported to have said, "Physicians are many in title but very few in number." I suspect that he alluded to the few who live up to his ideals, codified today in the Hippocratic Oath, and to the many who place personal lifestyle and financial enrichment ahead of service to their patients.

Roman philosopher Pliny the Elder (23–79), who once wrote that "true glory consists of doing what deserves to be written, and writing what deserves to be read," had this to say of physicians: "The medical profession is the only one in which anybody professing to be a physician is at once trusted, although nowhere else is an untruth more dangerous." I am fond of telling medical students that they can meet a patient for the first time and that person will tell the "student doctor" secrets he or she would not tell a mother. And then that newly met person will permit you to examine their body. This is all because you young and aspiring physicians inherit a legacy of trust that comes from the service, sacrifice, and honorable behavior of generations of physicians who preceded us. What legacy will you leave for the coming generations?

In the 16th century, Paracelsus wrote, "Every physician must be rich in knowledge, and not only of that which is written in books; his patients should be his book, they will never mislead him."

French novelist Honoré de Balzac (1799–1850) brings the creative writer's perspective in this quote: "The physician strives for the good as the artist strives for the beautiful, each pushed on by that admirable feeling we call virtue."

As we consider the character of the "true physician," German pathologist Rudolf Virchow (1821–1902) held that, "Only those who regard healing as the ultimate goal of their efforts can, therefore, be designated as physicians." And Irish/British playwright George Bernard Shaw (1856–1950) wrote in *The Doctor's Dilemma*: "But the true doctor is inspired by a hatred of ill-health, and a divine impatience of any waste of vital forces. Unless a man is led to medicine or surgery through a very exceptional aptitude, or because doctoring is a family tradition, or because he regards it unintelligently as a lucrative and gentlemanly profession, his motives in choosing the career of a healer are clearly generous" (5).

The Doctors Mayo—William James (1861–1939) and Charles Horace (1865–1939)—are best remembered as co-founders of the Mayo Clinic in Rochester, Minnesota. They were also the authors of numerous wise quotations: William, the elder of the two, tells us: "All who are benefited by community life, especially the physician, owe something to the community." Charles, the younger brother, said: "Physicians are not called or chosen; accident and environment brings about their choice of profession." He also wrote, "Given one well-trained [generalist] physician of the highest type he will do better work for a thousand people than ten specialists." The brothers Mayo died three months apart in 1939, and in 1964, were pictured on a 5-cent U.S. postage stamp.

American radiologist John L. McClenahan (1915–), who once wrote, "It requires a great deal of faith for a man to be cured by his own placebos," also offered this admonition: "It is because we have begun to act like merchants, and in many instances to observe the same hours, the public expects us to be regulated by the same restraints." This 1961 saying predated today's Nighthawk Radiology, a commercial venture in which roentgenograms taken in the early morning hours are read—via electronic transmission—by radiologists in India or Europe, who are in the middle of their workday. This allows the U.S. radiologist to observe a "9 to 5" professional lifestyle. You can purchase shares of Nighthawks Radiology Holdings, Inc., on the NASDAQ market; the ticker symbol is NHWK.

If young physicians could read just one paragraph about their chosen profession, I believe it should be "The Doctor," by Scottish writer Robert Louis Stevenson (1850–1894). As background, what you will read next was printed as a dedication in a book of poetry for children: *Underwoods: A Child's Garden of Verses* (6). It was written to thank, at the beginning of his book, "a few out of many doctors who have brought me comfort and help."

"There are men and classes of men that stand above the common herd; the soldier, the sailor, and the shepherd not infrequently; the artist rarely; rarely still, the clergyman; the physician almost as a rule. He is the flower (such as it is) of our civilization; and when that stage of man is done with, and only remembered to be marveled at in history, he will be thought to have shared as little as any in the defects of the period, and most notably exhibited the virtues of the race. Generosity he has, such as is possible to those who practice an art, never to those who drive a trade; discretion, tested by a hundred secrets; tact, tried in a thousand embarrassments; and what are more important, Heraclean cheerfulness and courage. So it is that he brings air and cheer into the sickroom, and often enough, though not so often as he wishes, brings healing."

Some Humorous Quotations About Medicine

Just so that we clinicians and scientists don't take ourselves too seriously, I will end the chapter with a few humorous sayings. If you enjoy the following, Brallier presents a good collection of witty sayings in his book *Medical Wit and Wisdom* (7).

- "Doctors are men who prescribe medicines of which they know little, to cure diseases of which they know less, in human beings of whom they know nothing." French philosopher François-Marie Arouet, aka Voltaire (1694–1778)
- "You [doctors] have, and always will be, exposed to the contempt of the gifted amateur—the gentleman who knows by intuition everything it has taken you years to learn." British author Rudyard Kipling (1865–1936)
- "The most tragic thing in the world is a sick doctor." Irish/British playwright George Bernard Shaw (1856–1950)
- "A hospital is no place to be sick." Polish-born American motion picture producer Samuel Goldwyn (1882–1974)
- "Never go to a doctor whose office plants have died." American humorist Erma Bombeck (1927–1996)

References

1. Dr. John Snow: a wonderful example of scientific thinking. Available at: http://www.physics.smu.edu/pseudo/DrSnow/. Accessed May 10, 2007.
2. O'Donnell M. *A Sceptic's Medical Dictionary*. London, UK: Blackwell BMJ Books; 1997.

3. Peabody FW. The care of the patient. *JAMA*. 1927;88:877–882.
4. Phillips WR, Haynes DG. The domain of family practice: scope, role, and function. *Fam Med*. 2001;33:273–277.
5. Shaw GB. *The Doctor's Dilemma*. Available at: http://www.gutenberg.org/etext/5070. Accessed May 14, 2007.
6. Stevenson RL. *Underwoods: A Child's Garden of Verses*. New York, NY: Peter Fenelon Collier & Son; 1887.
7. Brallier JM. *Medical Wit and Wisdom*. Philadelphia, PA: Running Press; 1993.

Part Three
Clinical Notes and
Medical Misadventures

9
Famous Persons as Patients

Health problems don't affect only so-called ordinary people; famous persons suffer illness, get hurt, occasionally experience physical or psychiatric impairment, and eventually breathe their last, just like the rest of us. Here are some examples: Earvin "Magic" Johnson has the human immunodeficiency virus (HIV); Ronald Reagan had Alzheimer disease; Annette Funicello has multiple sclerosis; Bob Dole suffered a right arm injury in World War II; Ray Charles was blind; actress Mary Tyler Moore is diabetic; and Albert Einstein may have had dyslexia.

The famous patients listed above as examples all had personal physicians. In a few instances, the physicians serving famous persons also become well known to the public. One example is President John F. Kennedy's personal physician, Dr. Janet Travell, who elucidated the role of trigger points in myofascial pain. She wrote her autobiography, *Office Hours, Day and Night* (1), and came to be called the "Mother of Myofascial Trigger Point Knowledge." You could add to the list the more infamous physicians (whose names I will not repeat here), who supplied drugs to Elvis Presley, Marilyn Monroe, and other celebrities. Most physicians to famous persons, however, remain more-or-less anonymous, caring for their noteworthy patients without themselves becoming famous for doing so.

My "famous patient" was world champion boxer Floyd Patterson (1935–2006), who was in my private practice when we both lived in the small town of New Paltz, New York, in the 1960s and 1970s. As happens often in a small town, Floyd and his family became friends of my family, and the association enriched our lives. Floyd died recently at his home, many years after I had moved to the West Coast.

Being Floyd Patterson's personal physician helped me understand that managing the health care of famous persons is not quite like treating persons who are not in the spotlight. Whenever Floyd and his family came to my office, there would be a "buzz" in the waiting room; strangers would go over to shake his hand. Sometimes, to protect his privacy, we would have him enter the office through the side door. Once Floyd suffered a hand laceration shortly before a major bout, necessitating a cancellation of an event that probably involved millions of dollars. As the treating physician, I was required to attest to the extent and severity of the injury. Later, when Floyd's last professional bout was stopped because Muhammad Ali opened a cut over Patterson's eye, I found myself late at night in a Manhattan hospital emergency room supervising the repair of the laceration. (There are techniques that should be used to ensure that the wound does not re-open when the area receives a blow in the future.)

I tell about my famous patient to highlight the facts that the illnesses and health care of noteworthy persons involve public curiosity, that what might seem a minor illness or injury can have far-reaching implications, and that occasionally your patient's health becomes entwined with events in history.

The very fact that all sick, injured, or disabled famous persons have personal physicians raises some interesting questions. First, does the very fact that the patient is "famous" change the medical care provided, and, if so, is fame—and often wealth—associated with better care or worse?

Illnesses of Noteworthy Persons

In discussing health issues of persons whose names we (should) all recognize, we sometimes can identify the illness with considerable certainty. Occasionally, we cross the line into probability. Then there is a thriving enterprise, sometimes called pathography, involved in postulating how disease might have influenced a person or a group at some point in history—an intriguing undertaking that we will visit later in the chapter.

Gout

U.S. statesman Benjamin Franklin was well known to have suffered gout. During one incapacitating gouty episode, he wrote two bagatelles (*The Deformed and Handsome Leg* and *Dialogue Between the Gout and Mr. Franklin*), which he sent to his neighbor Madame Brillon (2). During the same era, fellow gout sufferers were William Pitt, the Elder (1708–1778), as well as George Mason (1705–1792), John Hancock (1737–1792), Alexander Hamilton (1755–1804), and Thomas Jefferson (1743–1826). There seems to have been an "epidemic" of gout among America's Founding Fathers. Just to highlight that few adults have one single illness, Jefferson also suffered from headaches as well as lichen simplex chronicus and would pinch his skin and count to 10 to postpone scratching.

Other gout sufferers include French futurist Nostradamus (1503–1566), French theologian John Calvin (1509–1564), English poet John Milton (1608–1674), English physicist Sir Isaac Newton (1643–1727), Flemish artist Peter Paul Rubens (1577–1640), British monarch Queen Anne (1665–1714), English poet Alfred Lord Tennyson (1809–1892), German socialist revolutionary Karl Marx (1818–1883), and American movie actor-producer Mel Brooks (born 1926).

Agoraphobia

The word comes from ancient Greek words *agora* and *phobos* and literally means "fear of the marketplace." When out of their personal comfort zones, agoraphobics suffer severe anxiety and often panic attacks. Eventually, many cut off outside social contact and become housebound.

One apparent victim of agoraphobia was French mathematician and philosopher Blaise Pascal (1623–1662), who also suffered migraine headaches, as discussed later in the chapter. Another suspected victim was English naturalist Charles Darwin (1809–1882), remembered for his observations on the Galapagos Islands which led to his conception of evolution through natural selection, who probably suffered panic attacks and agoraphobia (3).

America's fourth president, James Madison (1751–1836), sometimes called the "Father of the Constitution," went to great lengths to avoid crowds and feared speaking in public.

Some famous actors are reported to have suffered agoraphobia. These include Woody Allen, Barbra Streisand, Kim Basinger, and Donny Osmond.

Huntington Disease

Named for American physician George Huntington (1850–1916) (see chapter 5), Huntington disease is a rare, inherited neurological disorder causing choreiform movements which typically begins in mid-life. Cognitive and psychiatric manifestations are common.

The disease might today be relegated to the obscurity of Morgellon disease or Jumping Frenchmen of Maine syndrome (see chapter 10) were it not for one man whose life and career were cut short by Huntington disease. Woody Guthrie (1912–1967) was born in Okemah, Oklahoma, which Guthrie would later describe as "one of the singingest, square dancingest, drinkingest, yellingest, preachingest, walkingest, talkingest, laughingest, cryingest, shootingest, fist fightingest, bleedingest, gamblingest, gun, club and razor carryingest of our ranch towns and farm towns" (4).

Guthrie was a folksinger who lived through the 1930s Dust Bowl years in the Great Plains. In 1941, Guthrie spent a month in Oregon working for the federal government, writing on contract a collection of songs intended to convince the public of the merits of placing dams on the Columbia River. One of these songs we all know is "Roll On, Columbia." Also, in the 1940s, he joined Pete Seeger and a politically active singing group in Greenwich Village, New York, called the Almanac Singers, which would later become the Weavers. You may recall the Weavers' hit song "Goodnight, Irene."

At the height of his career, Guthrie developed Huntington disease, and from 1954 until his death in 1967, he was repeatedly hospitalized for his illness. Following his death, his wife, Marjorie, created the Committee to

Combat Huntington's Disease, now called the Huntington Disease Society of America.

Recently, I drove along the gorge of the Columbia River while playing my CD of Guthrie's *Columbia River Suite*, a collection of his songs of the river recorded in his own voice, and I wondered what direction his career would have taken if not for his errant gene.

Depression and Bipolar Disorder

Now I will move from the uncommon illness to the very common—depression and bipolar disorder. One noteworthy person with depression was British statesman Sir Winston Churchill (1874–1965). Churchill suffered recurrent bouts of depression, which he described with the metaphor "my black dog." Storr has raised some interesting theories concerning Churchill, his "black dog," and the events of the mid-20th century. Young Winston spent much of his childhood at boarding schools, and hence his relationship with his parents was somewhat distant. Storr postulates a relationship between a depressive tendency and a sense of feeling unloved. A logical consequence was the emergence of the ambition to lead, i.e., "If I can't be loved, I'll find a way to be admired" (5).

The passionate, if compensatory, quest for leadership success may lead to great deeds, actually accomplished or sometimes merely attempted. And accidents of history may become major determinants. As it happened, Churchill reached the prime of his career just when he was most needed by the world, at the time that civilization was threatened by the Nazi menace. Storr asserts, "Only a man convinced that he had a heroic mission, who believed that, in spite of all evidence to the contrary, he could yet triumph, and who could identify himself with a nation's destiny could have conveyed his inspiration to others" (5).

Of course, feeling unloved can breed hostility, and what better target for hostility than Adolf Hitler and his Nazi storm troopers. Perhaps Churchill's depressive nature and his feelings of being unloved helped shape the character of the man who in 1940 would say, ". . . we shall fight on the beaches, we shall fight on the landing grounds, we shall fight in the fields and in the streets, we shall fight in the hills; we shall never surrender . . ."

As one who suffered depression, Churchill was in austere company. German composer Ludwig van Beethoven (1770–1827), in addition to being deaf, suffered bouts of manic depression, and like so many depressed persons, sometimes considered suicide. Bipolar mood swings may also have helped fuel the creative works of Charles Dickens (1812–1870) and Vincent van Gogh (1853–1890). The disease can reasonably be blamed for van Gogh's suicide at age 37.

Depression is sometimes called "the common cold of mental illness." The following is a list of well-known persons who are reported to have suffered from depression or bipolar disorder:

Menachem Begin, Prime Minister of Israel
Irving Berlin, composer
Marlon Brando, actor
Truman Capote, writer
Stan Getz, musician
Judy Garland, actress
Alexander Hamilton, politician
Stephen Hawking, physicist
Ernest Hemingway, author
Victor Hugo, author
Henrik Ibsen, playwright
Marilyn Monroe, actress
Georgia O'Keeffe, painter
George Patton, soldier
Edgar Allan Poe, author
Sylvia Plath, poet
Ezra Pound, poet
Percy Bysshe Shelley, poet
Pyotr (Peter) Ilyich Tchaikovsky, composer
Spencer Tracy, actor
Mark Twain, author
William Carlos Williams, physician and author
Natalie Wood, actress
Émile Zola, author

Epilepsy

Epilepsy is historically special in two ways. First of all, the defining disease manifestation—the seizure—is sufficiently recognizable that we can, with reasonable confidence, accept tales of historical figures reported to have epilepsy. Second, there is a long-standing and deep-rooted belief that epilepsy is somehow linked to genius. The epilepsy-genius assertion may not be quite as far-fetched as we evidence-based physicians would surmise, and the theory has its advocates. One of these is LaPlante, who believes that abnormal cortical activity noted in temporal lobe epilepsy is related to creative thinking and artistic inventiveness (6).

The connection between epilepsy and mystical powers might be traced to the time of Alexander the Great (356–323 BCE) (7). Alexander, aka Alexander III, King of Macedonia, had epilepsy. His illness did not prevent him from leading his armies to conquer most of the known world before his death at age 33. Other great leaders with epilepsy were Roman emperor Julius Caesar (100–44 BCE), whose seizures near the end of his life may have been caused by a brain tumor, and later Napoleon Bonaparte, Emperor of the French (1769–1821).

English poet Alfred Lord Tennyson (1809–1892) suffered "walking trances" as a youth and was subsequently diagnosed as epileptic. Tennyson saw his seizures as mystic visions, involving a loss of the sense of self.

Charles Dickens not only had epilepsy, he also described the disease in several characters in his books.

Vincent van Gogh, mentioned above as suffering from bipolar disorder, also had epileptic seizures, which he described as "the storm within." His best work—his paintings *Wheatfield with Crows*, *The Starry Night*, and his self-portraits—have been ascribed to the time of his greatest problems with seizures (7). Later in the chapter, I will tell you about a theory regarding how a side effect of van Gogh's epilepsy therapy just might be reflected in paintings we can view today.

Parkinson Disease

Just as epilepsy is—just possibly—associated with creative genius, Parkinson disease (PD) has been linked to high-achieving, well-known persons. In fact, the PD and fame link seems to be so strong that an essay on the Web site of the National Parkinson Foundation (NPF) asks, "Do famous people get PD more than ordinary people? Is there something about PD that first leads to fame, then PD?" (8). The Foundation Web site essay goes on to point out that PD affects 0.3% of Americans. Keep in mind that number as you consider that between 1927 and 2001, 49 different persons (a few persons were honored more than once) have been designated *Time* magazine's "Person of the Year." Three of these 49 individuals—Adolf Hitler, Deng Xiaoping, and Pope John Paul II—had PD. Three is 6% of 49, which is 20 times the prevalence in the U.S. population.

PD is a disease of maturity, with a peak onset at approximately age 60 years. Generally, PD lies dormant while its victim achieves success in life, and then reveals itself. Does this fact explain PD's apparently lofty prevalence among high achievers? The essay on the NPF Web site asks, "Or do famous people get PD because the brain, unknowingly, makes a Faustian bargain? Fame first—and then PD? Is there something about PD that leads to fame? Something that energized the brain before slowing it down? A 'slow-motion' form of bipolar disorder?"

Here are a few of the famous persons with PD:

Jack Anderson, newspaper columnist
Jim Backus, actor
Johnny Cash, singer
Salvador Dalí, artist
Billy Graham, evangelist
Katharine Hepburn, actress
Douglas MacArthur, American general
Janet Reno, U.S. attorney general
Terry-Thomas, British actor
Harry Truman, U.S. president

The caprice of research funding for a disease often depends on what famous persons have the disease. PD researchers and patients currently enjoy abundant funding thanks to two well-known and respected individuals who both contracted the disease when relatively young and who both are still living. The first was Muhammad Ali, who on September 20, 1972, opened the cut over the eye of my friend and patient Floyd Patterson; Ali's diagnosis of PD was made in 1991, when he was age 49. The second was actor Michael J. Fox, whose symptoms began at age 30. Fox writes of his disease in an autobiography entitled *Lucky Man*, and because of the heightened awareness his—and Muhammad Ali's—celebrity has brought to the disease, those searching for a way to prevent or cure PD have also experienced a little "luck."

Alzheimer Disease

While patients with epilepsy and PD can make televised appearances and help others by raising awareness of their illnesses, patients with Alzheimer disease (AD) seldom appear in public. Their degenerative neurologic disease destroys memory and impairs cognitive function, making public appearances problematic.

When we think of AD, many of us will think first of Ronald Reagan (1911–2004). At age 69, Reagan was elected the 40th president of the United States, the oldest person ever elected to the office. He had an engaging and persuasive style, earning him the sobriquet "the great communicator." Reagan and his wife, Nancy, called attention to the condition, and in conjunction with the Alzheimer's Association, founded the Ronald and Nancy Reagan Research Institute to help seek a way to prevent or cure the disease.

Some well-known actors and actresses have suffered AD. These include 1940s Hollywood pinup Rita Hayworth (1918–1987), movie "tough guy" Charles Bronson (1921–2003), and cinema hero-turned-political activist Charlton Heston (born 1924).

The list of persons with AD later in life includes several professional boxers, notably Sugar Ray Robinson (1921–1989) and Floyd Patterson. I believe that in these instances the problem was probably the long-term result of traumatic brain injury, rather than the garden-variety AD that afflicts many older persons.

Like Parkinson disease, AD typically begins in late life, after career goals have been achieved. For this reason, the list of famous persons with AD contains some familiar names:

> Dana Andrews, actor
> Imogene Coca, comedienne
> Ralph Waldo Emerson, author and philosopher
> Barry Goldwater, U.S. senator
> Jack Lord, actor
> Burgess Meredith, actor
> Rosa Parks, civil rights activist
> Joseph-Maurice Ravel, French composer
> Margaret Rutherford, British actress
> Robert Sargent Shriver, American politician

Migraine Headache

Migraine is a headache, generally one-sided and throbbing, that in its classic form is distinguished by an aura that precedes the pain and is characteristically associated with visual manifestations. The patient may describe zigzag lines (aka teichopsia), scintillating spots of light, scotomatous field cuts, or distorted visual perceptions. In fact, most migraineurs do not have the aura, but about one fourth of them do, and these persons can have some very interesting variations.

For example, French mathematician and philosopher Blaise Pascal left us clues to his migraine auras. On a few of Pascal's handwritten manuscript pages are crescent-shaped blank spots, just the shape of a scotoma. We can imagine Pascal busily writing when he has the onset of an aura with a blind spot. The pain is not present yet; that will come later. And so he hurriedly continues writing, ignoring the sections of the pages lost in the scotomatous void. Then, as he stops to think, he doodles zigzag lines in the margins of the manuscript.

Lewis Carroll (1832–1898) was a migraineur, and recognizing that I may be straying into retrospective diagnosis, some believe that the imagery of Carroll's work can be attributed to visual distortions experienced during the migraine aura. Those who examine his illustrations for *Alice's Adventures in Wonderland* and *Through the Looking-Glass* might note some zigzag patterns reminiscent of teichopsia. Carroll's contribution to medical imagery is also reflected in Alice in Wonderland syndrome, a rare type of migraine aura characterized by metamorphopsia—a perceptional distortion of visual image and perspective that the migraineur knows is not real.

French painter Georges-Pierre Seurat (1859–1891), a guiding light of the French school of neo-impressionism in the late 19th century, is remembered for his technique called pointillism, which creates images using very small dots ("points") of color. Today, the phenomenon of scintillating scotomata, which would describe small bright points of color or light, is called the "Seurat effect."

Spanish novelist and poet Miguel de Cervantes (1547–1616) was a migraineur. As he conceived of the windmills and other images we find in *Don Quixote de la Mancha*, might he have been influenced by a migraine aura with metamorphopsia?

I found no formal record that Spanish painter Pablo Picasso (1881–1973) suffered migraine headaches, but might he have had acephalgic migraine—migraine with aura, but without headache? Certainly Picasso's cubist paintings are reminiscent of visual distortions that some migraineurs describe as part of the aura.

Of course, not all migraineurs have entertaining visual phenomena. Most simply suffer their headaches, which can disrupt daily life. Sigmund Freud (1856–1939) tended to have migraines on Sundays. He called them his "weekend headaches," and good psychoanalyst that he was, he theorized that his feelings about anti-Semitism and the "Christian Sabbath" were responsible for the headaches.

U.S. president Thomas Jefferson (1743–1826) described a migraine episode in a letter to a friend: "... an attack of the periodical headache, which came on me about a week ago rendering me unable as yet either to write or read without great pain" (Strauss, p. 199).

Both leading generals of the U.S. Civil war—Robert E. Lee (1807–1870) and Ulysses S. Grant (1822–1885) suffered migraine headaches. So did Mary Todd Lincoln (1818–1882); her husband, the president, had his own health problems, which I will describe shortly.

Other noteworthy migraineurs in history include:

> Julius Caesar, Roman emperor
> Frédéric Chopin, Polish composer
> St. Luke, the physician
> Friedrich Nietzsche, German philosopher
> Alfred Nobel, Swedish manufacturer and inventor of dynamite
> Pyotr (Peter) Ilyich Tchaikovsky, Russian composer
> Leo Tolstoy, Russian philosopher and novelist
> Mary Tudor, Queen of England
> Virginia Woolf, British novelist

Diabetes Mellitus

Until 1922 (see chapter 1), a diagnosis of diabetes mellitus was a death sentence. With nothing but strict dietary measures to counter the hyperglycemia and inevitable acidosis, persons with type 1 diabetes (previously called "juvenile diabetes") often died young, before they achieved life goals and the chance to become famous. Hence, in history, the list of notable persons who both achieved fame and had diabetes is short.

The following is a list of some noteworthy diabetics. Note that all have lived since 1922.

> Arthur Ashe, professional tennis player
> Menachem Begin, Israeli prime minister
> Chris Dudley, professional basketball player
> Ella Fitzgerald, American jazz singer
> Mikhail Gorbachev, General secretary of the Communist Party of the Soviet Union
> Ray Kroc, American business leader (think McDonald's hamburgers)
> Marcello Mastroianni, Italian actor
> Mario Puzo, American novelist
> Kate Smith, American singer
> Jane Wyman, American actress

Seven percent of Americans have diabetes (9). Nevertheless, the disease is not in the public consciousness to quite the same degree as some other illnesses with more visible manifestations. Persons with diabetes do not fall to the floor with seizures. They do not develop tremors or lose their memories. In contrast to migraineurs, there are no legendary diabetics whose creativity can be traced to an episodic event. There is no lore linking diabetes to high achievement, as there is with PD. Diabetics simply struggle with their blood sugar levels and often, in the end, suffer premature atherosclerosis, peripheral neuropathy, renal failure, blindness, coronary artery disease, and early death.

Things are changing as more and more well-known persons with diabetes tell of their illness and lend their support to raising public awareness. A few current figures who do so are actresses Mary Tyler Moore and Halle Berry and professional basketball player Chris Dudley.

Breast Cancer

A tale of diseases of famous persons would be incomplete without a discussion of cancer, the second leading cause of death in the U.S. I have selected breast cancer as an example because the disease is very common; depending on whose statistics you read, 1 in every 7 to 10 U.S. women will develop breast cancer during her lifetime. Also, the disease can strike younger women during their most productive adult years; up to half of all cases begin in women under the age of 65.

Here are some noteworthy women reported to have had breast cancer (10):

> Brigitte Bardot, French actress and animal rights activist
> Linda Ellerbee, television journalist
> Peggy Fleming, Olympic figure skater
> Ann Jillian, actress
> Joan Kennedy, former wife of Senator Edward M. Kennedy
> Olivia Newton-John, Australian singer and actress
> Sandra Day O'Connor, Supreme Court Justice
> Nancy Reagan, former U.S. First Lady
> Suzanne Somers, actress
> Gloria Steinem, feminist activist

Just to keep in mind that approximately 1 percent of breast cancers occur in males, the list contains the names of two male breast cancer victims (10):

> Edward Brooke, former U.S. senator
> Richard Roundtree, actor

Examining the Heath of U.S. Presidents

History and the Health of Leaders

Over the past two centuries, the office of the president of the United States has become the most powerful position in the world. If we are to consider any series of famous patients, we must consider the health of America's leaders and sometimes look at how their health has affected the nation. It is a truism that presidents get sick, too. Furthermore, as prominent leaders, often surrounded by controversy, they are always potential targets for violence.

As we review selected U.S. presidents and their illnesses and injuries, think about how often America's first citizens received less than optimum care, owing to poor decisions, dithering, and meddling by so-called experts. Consider also the misinformation and secrecy that have sometimes attended presidential illness.

Selected U.S. Presidents: Their Illnesses and Injuries

George Washington (1732–1799)

Our first president was a hypochondriac. Perhaps he was influenced by the "family tradition of short-lived males" (11). For example, in 1752, his older half-brother, Lawrence, died early of tuberculosis. Lawrence plays a role in the drama because in 1751, George accompanied him as he sought a tropical environment to relieve his tubercular symptoms; their journeys took them to the island of Barbados, where George contracted smallpox. Fortunately surviving the disease, Washington bore both the facial scars for life and immunity to one of the diseases that threatened the Continental Army later in his career (11) (see chapter 2).

Washington's concern with his health continued until the end of his life. Moses and Cross report that he "predicted year after year that he would not live until his next birthday" (12). In the end, he died at age 67 while taking his own pulse. The cause of death was probably epiglottitis, along with the effects of heroic therapeutic bleeding, as discussed in chapter 11.

Thomas Jefferson (1743–1826)

As noted above, Jefferson had recurrent headaches and a chronic pruritic skin disease. He also was acutely aware of a lisp, and for this reason, preferred writing to speaking. Perhaps this had something to do with his being the chief author of the United States Declaration of Independence.

Despite various illnesses, Jefferson had an aversion to physicians and declined medical attention if at all possible. For example, on one occasion, he fractured a wrist and refused medical care, preferring to accept the resulting deformity (12).

Andrew Jackson (1767–1845)

America's seventh president was called "Old Hickory" because of his sturdiness and personal forcefulness. It is thus a little surprising that he was arguably the most illness-ridden of our presidents, with no less than 10 items on his medical problem list. Jackson, like Washington, was a smallpox survivor. Like Jefferson, he suffered from a chronic pruritic skin disorder. His medical history includes various febrile illnesses, headaches, malaria, dysentery, toothaches, and partial blindness (13). He suffered a gunshot wound as a young man, and another in 1806. The latter gunshot was a chest wound, which resulted in a chronic lung infection. He died at age 78 of tuberculosis and heart failure.

William Henry Harrison (1773–1841)

The ninth president of the United States established several impressive records. At age 68, he was the oldest person ever elected to the office, a distinction held until the 1980 election of Ronald Reagan at age 69. Harrison's was the shortest presidential term in U.S. history, and he was the first U.S. president to die in office.

Harrison was inaugurated as president on March 4, 1841, enduring bitter cold weather without an overcoat and delivering the longest inaugural address in history—almost two hours in length, another presidential record that still stands. Harrison promptly developed a respiratory infection, culminating in pneumonia and death one month later, on April 4, 1841.

Abraham Lincoln (1809–1865)

The first president from the Republican Party, Lincoln held the nation together during the Civil War while serving as the 16th U.S. president. Two health issues have held our attention over the years. One is the speculation concerning the possibility that Lincoln had Marfan syndrome, which I will discuss in the next section of the chapter.

The other issue is Lincoln's tendency to suffer depressive episodes, which plagued him all his life. During his presidency, the "Great Emancipator" suffered recurrent, sometimes near-suicidal bouts of depression. In addition, Lincoln's other health issues included colorblindness, vertical strabismus, a deformity of the chest wall, bunions, and corns.

Grover Cleveland (1837–1908)

Grover Cleveland was both the 22nd and 24th president of the United States, the only president to serve two non-consecutive terms. In 1893, during his second term, Cleveland developed a sarcoma of the maxilla. Telling not even his wife, Cleveland secretly had the tumor removed during surgery aboard a colleague's yacht.

Woodrow Wilson (1856–1924)

Woodrow Wilson served as the 28th U.S. president from 1913 until 1921. Among his achievements, Wilson led America in "the War to Make the World Safe for Democracy." He was also the victim of one of the most serious instances of disability in a U.S. president. On October 2, 1919, Wilson suffered a stroke resulting in a left-sided hemiplegia and blindness in the left eye. He used a wheelchair at first but eventually could walk with the help of a cane, although presidential duties presented a great challenge. Wilson, his wife Edith, and their close associates decided to keep secret the extent of the president's disability. Edith became his "prime minister," determining what problems would be brought to her husband and managing the Cabinet and Congress until his term of office expired in 1921.

Franklin D. Roosevelt (1882–1945)

FDR was the 32nd U.S. president and the only president to serve more than two terms in office. His leadership of the nation began with the Great Depression and continued through World War II. In August 1921, Roosevelt contracted an illness, believed to be polio, that caused permanent paralysis of his lower body. From then on, Roosevelt labored to minimize his disability, especially in the eyes of the American people. He was careful not to be seen in public sitting in the wheelchair that he used in private. When making a public appearance, Roosevelt did his best to appear upright and mobile; he was able to stand with some support and he could walk using braces and a cane.

Later in life, Roosevelt developed another problem, hypertensive cardiovascular disease and heart failure, described in chapter 2 as an illness that influenced history. Roosevelt's severe hypertension—often exceeding 200/100 mm Hg—was diagnosed as early as March 1944. According to Ferrell, all involved—including his physicians—participated in a conspiracy of silence, keeping the facts of Roosevelt's precarious health from the Allies, from Vice President Harry S. Truman, and apparently from Roosevelt himself. Roosevelt's illness was also kept secret from the public, who reelected him president in November 1944 (14).

Dwight D. Eisenhower (1890–1969)

"Ike" became the 34th U.S. president after serving as Supreme Commander of the Allied Forces in Europe in World War II. He had two significant medical events during his time in office.

In September 1955, near the end of his first term of office, Eisenhower suffered a heart attack.

To calm the American public, experts of the day minimized the implications of a myocardial infarction, seeming to say that the president had suffered a minor illness. Then in June 1956, nine months following his heart attack, the 65-year-old president suffered an attack of regional enteritis, aka Crohn disease. The episode caused obstruction of the small bowel, necessitating surgery (15). Again the public was reassured.

In November 1956, Eisenhower was elected to a second term as president.

John F. Kennedy (1917–1963)

The 35th U.S. president, Jack Kennedy, came into office in 1961 with a medical secret. In 1947, Kennedy had been diagnosed with Addison disease, a deficiency of adrenal hormones. During the presidential campaign of 1960, rumors of Kennedy's adrenal deficiency began to surface. His personal physician, Dr. Janet Travell, explicitly denied the rumors, stating, "John F. Kennedy has not, nor has he ever, had . . . Addison's disease" (16).

The Addison disease secret was kept throughout Kennedy's presidency, although the rumors persisted. Photographs suggesting the possibility of steroid-induced facial swelling did not reassure the skeptics. And of course, the likelihood that Kennedy was taking steroids while in office brings to mind some of the side effects of corticosteroids, which include disturbances of mood or sleep and even hypomania or psychosis.

Eventually, other problems surfaced, including Kennedy's addiction to analgesics, presumably prescribed for his recurrent back pain. All ended with Kennedy's assassination in Dallas, Texas, on November 22, 1963.

Retrospective Diagnosis and Famous Persons

Through the Retrospectroscope

Retrospective diagnostic theorization is a thriving enterprise in the 21st century. Here is an example: We know from history that on March 1, 1953, a vigorous Joseph Stalin dined with friends, then collapsed with a stroke, probably hemorrhagic in nature; he died four days later. In 2003, a team of medical historians offered the opinion that Stalin had been poisoned with warfarin (see chapter 3), a flavorless anticoagulant that, taken in high doses, could very well cause a cerebral hemorrhage. The warfarin theory is intriguing and appears to be safe from factual refutation (17). I offer this story as an example of mining history to find previously unsuspected health issues in the lives of famous persons. Some more of these speculative tales follow.

Medical Reconsideration of Historical Events

King Tutankhamun (ca. 1358–1340 BCE)

In 1922, British Egyptologist Howard Carter, supported by his patron Lord Carnarvon, discovered the tomb of Tutankhamun in Egypt's Valley of the Kings near Luxor. Following the subsequent excavation, Carter and Lord Carvarvon entered the tomb three weeks later, and then on February 16, 1923, Carter first opened the burial chamber containing the sarcophagus.

"King Tut" began his reign at age 9 and died at age 18, which raises the question: "How did this young man die?" Could there have been foul play?

Or did he die of natural causes? A 1968 roentgenogram of the mummy revealed a dense area at the base of the skull, perhaps with some calcification present, indicating that there had been time for some healing to begin. The apparent answer was a blow to the skull causing a subdural hematoma that may have caused death, and Egyptologists promptly began the hunt for a perpetrator, such as Tut's immediate successor, Ay.

Then, with advances in technology, a computed tomography (CT) scan of the mummy revealed that there actually was a hole in the head—presumably drilled by ancient embalmers. The CT scan also revealed a severe leg fracture, leading to the conclusion that the prince had died of gangrene that followed the broken leg. The scan revealed no evidence of a blow to the head, ending the "murder investigation."

King David the Great of Israel (ca. 1011–971 BCE)

Toward the end of his life, King David, the second and greatest king of Israel, suffered progressive anorexia, weight loss, and eventual cachexia. Biblical passages include ". . . I forgot to eat my bread" and ". . . my bones cleave to my skin." Scholars have searched the Bible for clues and speculated regarding the cause of the king's deterioration. Ben-Noun suggests several possibilities, of which two seem likely suspects: The first is depression, compounded by the social isolation of being a king, leading to profound anorexia. The second possibility is carcinoma of the prostate or other organ, with metastasis to the bones (18).

St. Paul of Tarsus (ca. 3–62 CE)

Paul of Tarsus, aka Paul the Apostle, was a leader in spreading Christianity beyond Israel. His conversion to Christianity came during an experience on the fabled road to Damascus. Paul suddenly experienced a bright light and fell to the ground, temporarily blinded. Scholars have debated the various physiologic explanations. The most plausible seems to be that Paul suffered temporal lobe epilepsy with ecstatic seizures.

Temporal lobe epilepsy with ecstatic seizures is also called Dostoevsky epilepsy. In his novel *The Idiot*, Russian novelist and known epileptic Fyodor Dostoevsky (1821–1881) depicted this type of seizure in his character Prince Myshkin (19).

"He remembered that during his epileptic fits, or rather immediately preceding them, he had always experienced a moment or two when his whole heart, and mind and body seemed to wake up with vigor and light. . . . Next moment something appeared to burst open before him; a wonderful inner light illuminated his soul. This lasted perhaps a second, yet he distinctly remembered hearing the beginning of a wail, the strange dreadful wail, which bursts from his lips of its own accord, and which no effort of will on his part could suppress. Next moment he was absolutely unconscious; black darkness blotted out everything. He had fallen in an epileptic fit."

Joan of Arc (1412–1431)

The uneducated young woman from a rural French village who inspired historic military victories seemed to have had ecstatic experiences, not unlike those of St. Paul of Tarsus. In addition, her femininity has been the subject of anachronistic scrutiny. Greenblatt has suggested that, based on various reports of her life and her appearance, Joan suffered from androgen insensitivity syndrome, previously called the testicular feminization syndrome. Reports from her time indicate that Joan was a well-developed peasant girl with a feminine voice, normal breast development, absence of pubic hair, and amenorrhea—a reasonable description of the manifestations of androgen insensitivity syndrome (20).

If all the above is true, then Joan had not one, but two diseases: temporal lobe epilepsy with ecstatic seizures and also androgen insensitivity syndrome.

Ivan IV, First Tzar of Russia (1530–1584)

Ivan IV, whom we recall as Ivan the Terrible, was crowned Tzar in 1547, at the age of 17. In that same year, he married Anastasia Zakharina-Koshkina. In his early years as leader of Russia, he ruled about as wisely as his contemporary heads of state—involved in the affairs of government, available to his subjects, and yet sometimes cruel. But much worse was to come.

We believe today that Ivan IV contracted syphilis sometime before his marriage in 1547. In 1552, the first son of the royal couple died at age 6 weeks, possibly of congenital syphilis. Their third son, Fedor, was probably a congenital syphilitic.

Ivan's reign of terror followed the death of Anastasia in 1560. Floggings, boilings, and other hideous deaths alternated with devout prayer. Thousands died. In the end, Ivan killed his own son and heir, Tzarevitch Ivan. The change is his personality and the events recorded are considered evidence that Ivan IV "was suffering from cerebral syphilis" (Cartwright, p. 67).

Ironically, syphilis was perhaps not Ivan's cause of death. An examination of the Tzar's remains in the 1960s revealed toxic levels of mercury in the tissues, suggesting that perhaps those about him had despaired of his insane cruelty and had poisoned him.

King George III of England (1738–1820)

King George III ruled before and during the American Revolution. Few would disagree that George III's ill treatment of the American colonists and his subsequent mismanagement of the Revolutionary War were major factors in establishing an independent United States of America.

During his reign, some of the decisions of George III were highly illogical. At times he seemed mad, so much so that Parliament debated his fitness to wear the crown. Ellis reports one rumor of the time that "George III's mounting insanity had produced a delusional fit in which he imagined himself to be the second coming of [George] Washington" (p. 184).

In the 1960s, Macalpine and Hunter advanced the theory that George III may have had a type of porphyria. Physician notes of the time indicate that, in addition to his "madness," George III suffered abdominal pain, constipation, weakness in the extremities, and dark, reddish urine. The authors support their case by tracing porphyria back to George III's ancestor Mary Queen of Scots and forward to his descendant Queen Anne, the last Stuart monarch (21). An aggravating factor may have been King George's consumption of lead-containing Portuguese wine.

Not all experts agree with Macalpine and Hunter, but the theory is well established in the public consciousness, especially since the release of the 1994 motion picture *The Madness of King George*.

Napoleon Bonaparte (1769–1821)

During his reign, Napoleon Bonaparte, Emperor of the French, came to control most of continental Europe; some nations were conquered, others joined in alliances with the powerful French monarch. In the end, Napoleon was defeated in 1815 by the British at the Battle of Waterloo, in Belgium. Later that year, he was exiled to the bleak island of St. Helena, where he died in 1821.

Historians have long attributed Napoleon's death to stomach cancer, an illness that had afflicted several members of his family. However, Forshufvud has suggested that Napoleon died of arsenic poisoning (22). Napoleon's health declined rapidly beginning only a few months before his death at age 52. Symptoms included headache, photophobia, rapid pulse, gastrointestinal complaints, swollen feet, and alternating insomnia and somnolence. These symptoms are all consistent with arsenic poisoning, but are by no means diagnostic.

It seems that, following Napoleon's death, his valet shaved the scalp, and the hairs were saved. Later analysis of the scalp hair has revealed a very high level of arsenic.

An odd clincher may be as follows: In 1840, when Napoleon's body was exhumed for transportation to France, his remains were noted to be unusually well preserved. One compound that can inhibit the enzymes of decomposition is arsenic (23).

Meriwether Lewis (1777–1809)

Napoleon sold the Louisiana Territory to Thomas Jefferson and the United States in 1803. In 1804, Jefferson dispatched Captain Meriwether Lewis, private secretary to the president, and Second Lieutenant William Clark to explore the new purchase. The journey lasted from May 14, 1804, until the "Corps of Discovery" arrived at St. Louis, Missouri, on September 23, 1806.

On October 11, 1809, Lewis died at a tavern near Nashville, Tennessee, while en route to Washington. The cause of death was a gunshot wound. The question arises: Was he killed or was his death a suicide?

Reports surrounding the incident indicate that Lewis had been severely depressed, even attempting to kill himself by drowning in the Mississippi River not long before the fatal event. To help shed light on the mystery, Westefeld uses a risk factor model for suicide assessment "to evaluate the nature of Lewis' historical, personal, psychosocial, environmental, and clinical risk factors and protective factors." The conclusion is that "the preponderance of the evidence indicates that he died by his own hand" (24).

Only one small question remains: Lewis was shot in both the head and the chest. Lewis was a soldier, very familiar with firearms. If a suicide, is it not likely that he would have required only one shot?

Abraham Lincoln (1809–1865)

Did the 16th president of the United States have Marfan syndrome, or did he not? Even if he did not, Lincoln's general appearance has helped many aspiring physicians recall the autosomal dominant connective tissue disorder characterized by very long arms and legs, hypermobility of joints, arachnodactyly, ectopia lentis, pectus carinatum, thoracic aneurysm, aortic regurgitation, and mitral valve prolapse. As a clinical pearl, Ellerin and Diaz state, "If the outstretched arm length is greater than the patient's height, suspect Marfan syndrome" (p. 13).

For more than 40 years, physicians and medical historians have debated whether Lincoln had Marfan syndrome. Advocates of the theory cite his great height, long limbs, and apparently lax joints. Skeptics cite Lincoln's well-recognized physical strength, allowing him to perform feats of strength, such as holding a heavy ax at arm's length by the tip of the handle, a feat unlikely to be accomplished by a patient with the connective tissue defects of Marfan syndrome. In addition, the retrospective diagnosis seems to be chiefly based on Lincoln's body habitus, without the collaboration of ocular, cardiac, or vascular findings (25).

Charles Darwin (1809–1882)

The English naturalist who proposed that evolutionary change occurs through natural selection suffered for decades with symptoms of abdominal pain, vomiting, fatigue, and headache. Many theories have been advanced in efforts to explain Darwin's illness, including hypochondria, psychophysiologic causes, and the ever-popular arsenic poisoning.

In 2005, Campbell and Matthews proposed a new theory, that Darwin's illness was caused by lactose intolerance. They report, "Vomiting and gut problems showed up two to three hours after a meal, the time it takes for lactose to reach the large intestine. His family shows a major inherited component, as with genetically disposed hypolactasia. Darwin only got better when, by chance, he stopped taking milk and cream" (26).

Florence Nightingale (1820–1910)

"The Lady with the Lamp" was the founder of nursing as we know it today. Her best-known achievements took place during her service in the Crimean War (1854–1857), after which she returned to England and suffered a variety of symptoms which often caused her to be bedridden, believing she might die at any moment.

At age 16, Nightingale, a very religious person, experienced a supernatural call to help the suffering, which led to her career in nursing. Her illness began when she was a young woman, with fever, weakness, palpitations, spinal pain, and nervous tremors. During her middle years, she worked tirelessly, almost urgently, while she suffered headaches, insomnia, and depression with feelings of worthlessness. Later in life, her symptoms seemed to abate, and she died at age 90 of heart failure.

Many have debated the origin of Nightingale's symptoms and her ability to be highly productive in the face of apparent illness. Some have suggested chronic brucellosis as the underlying malady. Others have suggested feigned illness with "strategic invalidism." Wisner et al. postulate, "I submit that our patient had bipolar disorder with psychotic features" (27). They cite the age of onset of the symptoms, the characteristics of her depressed phases, her "mystical experiences," and partial relief obtained late in life.

Whatever her malady, she remains honored for her contributions to compassionate patient care, professionalism in hospital management, and a scholarly and statistically oriented approach to the study of health care delivery.

Vincent van Gogh (1853–1890)

Here I return to van Gogh. During his later years, the Dutch Postimpressionist's paintings are noteworthy for yellow tones and halos, characteristics that have been attributed to visual causes such as glaucoma, cataracts, and solar injury. The painter's lusty consumption of absinthe may have played a role.

In 1981, Lee proposed a medically credible hypothesis: digitalis intoxication (28). As mentioned above, van Gogh had epilepsy, a disease that at the end of the 19th century was often treated with digitalis. Two of the manifestations of digitalis intoxication are xanthopsia (yellow vision) and visual coronas. Collaborating evidence of the theory is that the artist twice depicted his physician in paintings holding a foxglove plant—just as if van Gogh were leaving a clue for posterity.

William Howard Taft (1857–1930)

America's 27th president was a huge man, weighing up to 340 pounds. He once became stuck in the White House bathtub. His tendency to fall asleep at unlikely times was legendary. As suggested by Sotos, Taft's daytime somnolence, hypertension, and perhaps even "cognitive and psychosocial impairment" seem to justify a diagnosis of sleep apnea (29). In fact, the symptoms seem pickwickian (see chapter 5).

The diagnostic presumption is reinforced by reports that, following the loss of 60 pounds, Taft's somnolence resolved.

Albert Einstein (1879–1955)

Some consider theoretical physicist and Nobel Prize recipient Albert Einstein the foremost scientist in history. His work in formulating the general and special theories of relativity is evidence of his genius. Would you then be surprised to learn that he might have had attention deficit virgule hyperactivity disorder (ADHD)?

ADHD has traditionally been considered a childhood disorder, but recently it has become fashionable to make the diagnosis in adults—so-called adult ADHD. In a popular book, Hallowell and Ratey suggest that Einstein may have had ADHD (30). Despite a paucity of compelling evidence to support the theory, the mere association of Einstein's name with the disorder must be a small comfort to ADHD patients and families everywhere.

Franklin D. Roosevelt (1882–1945)

Here we return to FDR in the context of retrospective diagnosis. For decades, Americans have associated the 32nd President of the United States with poliomyelitis, which he contracted in 1921 at 39 years of age. It would not be unfair to say that Roosevelt became the public face of the disease. The image of his courageous struggle helped create and fund the March of Dimes and eventually the development of the Salk polio vaccine.

Today, there is speculation that Roosevelt did not have polio at all, but instead was a victim of Guillain-Barré syndrome. The age at onset and some features of Roosevelt's disease were always inconsistent with the classic picture of polio. Goldman et al. investigated the likelihood of the two diseases by means of Bayesian analysis, concluding that six of eight posterior probabilities (measurements of likelihood) strongly favor a diagnosis of Guillain-Barré syndrome for Roosevelt (31).

I wonder whether a diagnosis of Guillain-Barré syndrome instead of polio in 1921 would have affected the later fundraising that supported the development of the Salk vaccine.

If you would like to learn more about the illnesses of FDR and other famous persons and stories of the "celebritization of patienthood," I recommend Lerner's book, *When Illness Goes Public: Celebrity Patients and How We Look at Medicine* (32).

References

1. Travell JG. *Office Hours, Day and Night: The Autobiography of Janet Travell, MD*. New York, NY: World Publishing Co.; 1968.

2. The Papers of Benjamin Franklin. Available at: http://www.yale.edu/franklinpapers. Accessed May 16, 2007.
3. Barloon TJ, Noyes R Jr. Charles Darwin and panic disorder. *JAMA*. 1997;277:138–141.
4. Woody Guthrie biography. Available at: http://www.woodyguthrie.org/biography.htm. Accessed May 12, 2007.
5. Storr A. *Churchill's Black Dog, Kafka's Mice, and Other Phenomena of the Human Mind*. New York, NY: Grove Press; 1988.
6. LaPlante E. *Seized*. New York, NY: HarperCollins; 1993.
7. Famous People with Epilepsy. Available at: http://www.epilepsy.com/epilepsy/famous.html. Accessed May 16, 2007.
8. Fame and Parkinson disease. Available at: http://www.Parkinson.org. Accessed March 16, 2007.
9. Total prevalence of diabetes in the United States, all ages, 2005. Available at: http://diabetes.niddk.nih.gov/dm/pubs/statistics/index.htm#7. Accessed May 14, 2007.
10. List of notable breast cancer patients according to survival status. Available at: http://en.wikipedia.org/wiki/List_of_notable_breast_cancer_patients_according_to_survival_status. Accessed May 14, 2007.
11. Ellis JJ. *His Excellency: George Washington*. New York, NY: Knopf; 2005:8–9.
12. Moses JB, Cross W. Presidential medical quiz. *American Med News*. 1980; July 11:6.
13. Moses JB. *Presidential Courage*. New York, NY: Norton; 1980.
14. Ferrell RH. *The Dying President: Franklin D. Roosevelt, 1944–1945*. Columbia: University of Missouri Press; 1998.
15. Heaton LD, Ravdin IS, Blades B, Whelan TJ. President Eisenhower's operation for regional enteritis: a footnote to history. *Ann Surg*. 1964;159:661–666.
16. When the President is the Patient. Available at: http://www.healthmedialab.com/html/president/index.html. Accessed May 16, 2007.
17. Brent J, Naumov V. *Stalin's Last Crime: The Plot Against the Jewish Doctors, 1948–1953*. New York, NY: HarperCollins; 2003.
18. Ben-Noun LL. The disease that caused weight loss in King David the Great. *J Gerontol A Biol Sci Med Sci*. 2004;59:143–145.
19. Dostoevsky F. *The Idiot*. Originally published in 1869. Cited in: Temporal Lobe Epilepsy. Available at:http://www.epilepsy.com/epilepsy/epilepsy_temporallobe.html. Accessed May 14, 2007.
20. Greenblatt RB. Joan of Arc's amenorrhea. *Diagnosis*. 1983; March; 171–173.
21. Macalpine I, Hunter R. *George III and the Mad-Business*. London, UK: Allen Lane and the Penguin Press; 1969.
22. Forshufvud S. *Who Killed Napoleon?* London, UK: Hutchinson; 1962.
23. Weider B, Forshufvud S. *Assassination at St. Helena Revisited*. New York, NY: Wiley; 1995.
24. Westefeld JS, Less A. Meriwether Lewis: was it suicide? *Suicide Life Threat Behav*. 2004;34:220–227.
25. Holzer H. The health of Abraham Lincoln. *MD*. 1983; February:83–93.
26. Campbell AK, Matthews SB. Darwin's illness revealed. *Postgrad Med J*. 2005;81:248–251.
27. Wisner KL, Bostridge M, Mackowiak PA. A case of glimmering gloom. *Pharos Alpha Omega Alpha Honor Med Soc*. 2005 Autumn; 68:4–13.

28. Lee TC. Van Gogh's vision. Digitalis intoxication? *JAMA*. 1981;245:727–729.
29. Sotos JG. Taft and Pickwick: sleep apnea in the White House. *Chest*. 2003;124:1133–1142.
30. Hallowell EM, Ratey JJ. *Driven to Distraction: Recognizing and Coping with Attention Deficit Disorder*. New York, NY: Touchstone; 1994.
31. Goldman AS, Schmalstieg EJ, Freeman DH Jr., Goldman DA, Schmalstieg FC Jr. What was the cause of Franklin Delano Roosevelt's paralytic illness? *J Med Biogr*. 2003;11:232–240.
32. Lerner BH. *When Illness Goes Public: Celebrity Patients and How We Look at Medicine*. Baltimore, MD: Johns Hopkins University Press; 2006.

10
Short Tales of Serendipity, Curiosities, Medical Trivia, Authorship, and Speculation

This chapter is a potpourri of stories that touch on various aspects of medicine. Faced with the task of ordering them somehow, I have arranged them under five categories: **serendipity**, telling about some fortuitous advances in medicine; **curiosities**, describing a selection of fascinating clinical phenomena; **trivia**, telling some short stories about diseases, remedies, and persons; **authorship**, recording some little-known facts about medical reference books; and **speculation**, offering some theories about how disease just might possibly have influenced the world as we know it today.

Serendipity and Some Fortuitous Advances in Medicine

I will begin by confiding that I have always liked the word *serendipity* (along with *borborygmus* and *triskaidekaphobia*). As words go, *serendipity* is a relative newcomer, coined in 1754 by English physicist Horace Walpole and based on a Persian tale entitled *The Three Princes of Serendip*. Serendip is an ancient Persian name for Ceylon, later called Sri Lanka. The princes were blessed with a series of lucky findings. In Walpole's words, "As their highnesses traveled, they were always making discoveries by accident and sagacity, of things they were not in quest of" (1).

Serendipity seems to be the actualization of the chapter 1 quote from Louis Pasteur: "Chance only favors the prepared mind." For example, Isaac Newton (1643–1727) comes to mind. If we believe the oft-told tale, an apple falling from a tree inspired Newton to formulate the theory of universal gravitation. From chapter 1, we recall Fleming's discovery of penicillin, growing on a carelessly placed culture plate that luckily was not destroyed because of the contamination. A more recent instance is the story of a man walking in the countryside who found cockleburs clinging to his clothing; he went on to develop a fastening system called Velcro. The "vel" comes from *velvet*, the "cro" from the hooked needle used in crocheting (2). Another example is the Post-it note, which evolved from a failed endeavor to develop a strong adhesive; instead, the result was a weak adhesive, which might have been discarded had not a "prince of Serendip"' thought to use the adhesive to create bookmarks that would not damage pages. The following are some other examples of medical serendipity.

Cellini and Mercury as a Treatment for Syphilis

Weiss (pp. 5–7) tells the story of Florentine sculptor Benvenuto Cellini (1500–1571). Following an "indiscretion" with one of his models, Cellini developed syphilis, and there are historical clues that his disease progressed to involve the central nervous system. About this time, Cellini seems to have developed some business enemies, who poisoned the sculptor with mercury during a banquet. The patient's abdominal pain and bloody diarrhea convinced a physician of the diagnosis of mercury poisoning.

Following this episode, Cellini continued to be brilliantly productive and lived to age 71, neither likely in a man with progressive neurosyphilis. As Weiss concludes, "This whole episode is memorialized in Cellini's breathtaking larger-than-life bronze sculpture of the period, *Perseus with the Head of Medusa*. At the base of the statue, helping support the mythological hero and his trophy, Cellini placed a figure of the god Mercury flanked by representations of the multibreasted venereal goddess" (p. 7).

By including these figures at the base of the stature (now exhibited at the Loggia dei Lanzi gallery in Florence), Cellini seems to be sending the message that he knew of his serendipitous cure.

Hahnemann, Homeopathy, and Immunizations

Samuel Hahnemann (1755–1843), recalled today as the founder of homeopathic medicine, based his teachings on the theory that "like cures like." Homeopathy, an alternative to allopathic medicine, uses very small doses of compounds to treat disease.

Some of the doses were quite small—microdoses.

Hahnemann's homeopathy and its tiny doses of medication threatened the scientific tenets of both allopathic physicians and chemists (pharmacists) of his time, and both groups attacked his school of medicine. Today, there are practitioners of homeopathy in many countries worldwide, but the dominant ideology is clearly allopathic.

The advocates of "like cures like" in microdoses can be considered to have advanced medical thinking in one special way—immunizations. Hahnemann was a contemporary of Edward Jenner (1749–1823) and lived at a time when the medical world was becoming excited about "vaccination," using a small dose of a material to protect against a virulent disease. The use of microdoses of organisms to induce immunity and thereby prevent disease is a cornerstone of modern preventive medicine. In fact, immunizations against diseases such as diphtheria, tetanus, pertussis, measles, and so forth have arguably saved more lives than antimicrobials.

According to Inglis, Emil Adolf von Behring (1854–1917), winner of the 1901 Nobel Prize in Physiology or Medicine for developing a serum therapy against diphtheria and tetanus, credits Hahnemann with being a pioneer in immunizations: "In spite of all scientific speculations and experiments regarding smallpox vaccination, Jenner's discovery remained an erratic block in medicine, till the biochemical thinking Pasteur, devoid of all medical classroom knowledge, traced the origin of this therapeutic block to a principle which cannot better be characterized than by Hahnemann's word: Homeopathic" (quoted in Inglis, p. 125).

Hahnemann set out to *cure* "like" with "like," but in the end he serendipitously showed us the principle of *preventing* like with like.

Simpson and Chloroform Anesthesia

In 1831, Scottish professor of surgery James Young Simpson (1811–1870) was working with a group of assistants, testing various chemicals, one of which was chloroform. A bottle was opened in the room full of young persons as they continued their work. As the story goes, Simpson's wife later entered the room to bring in dinner only to find them all asleep. Simpson recognized the significance of his fortuitous discovery and next used chloroform to provide anesthesia to a woman in labor. He continued use in other patients and word of chloroform anesthesia spread.

As sometimes happens, a medical advance becomes popularized when a well-known person becomes an advocate. Chloroform gained recognition when used as anesthesia by Queen Victoria in 1853 as she was giving birth to Prince Leopold. By coincidence, the physician who administered the anesthesia to the Queen was John Snow (1813–1858), who aborted a cholera epidemic by his public health activism in 1854 (see chapter 1) (Porter, p. 367).

Soon thereafter, the chloroform anesthesia eclipsed the use of ether, which had proven effective but was attended by troublesome side effects. Simpson's recognition of the soporific qualities of chloroform led to a significant advance in surgical anesthesia.

Osler and His Move to America

In 1884, Sir William Osler (1849–1919) was in Leipzig, Germany, paying a visit to a colleague, pathologist Rudolf Virchow (1821–1902), remembered today with the eponymous Virchow node. During his sojourn, Osler received a message offering him the post of professor of medicine at the University of Pennsylvania in Philadelphia.

Already holding the position of professor of medicine at McGill University in Montreal, Osler was torn. Should he accept this new opportunity or should he stay with his colleagues in Canada? He decided to make his decision with the flip of a coin: heads, Philadelphia; tails, Montreal. The coin landed heads, and Osler was off to Philadelphia, later to move to Johns Hopkins University in Baltimore, Maryland. This was good fortune indeed for American medicine.

Halsted and Surgical Gloves

By 1889, word of Lister's 1866 antisepsis technique had spread to America. An early advocate was William S. Halsted, who had pioneered a number of surgical advances, including performing the first radical mastectomy for breast cancer.

Porter (p. 373) explains that, because of the noxious fumes of Lister's carbolic acid, Halsted was relegated to performing his surgery not in the operating room, but in the marquees in the garden of New York Bellevue Hospital. But this is not the remarkable part of the tale. Nor is the fact that Halsted initially used protective rubber gloves in the dissection room, but not during surgery.

As it happened, Halsted was engaged to marry Caroline Hampton, his surgical nurse. His fiancée complained that the chemical disinfectant caused severe dermatitis of her hands. Halsted persuaded the Goodyear Rubber Company to manufacture thin rubber gloves that would protect Caroline's hands, but not interfere with sensitive touch. Caroline wore the newly invented surgical gloves; Halsted did not, at least at first. In time, he came to recognize their value in antisepsis, an unexpected outcome of his quest to protect the skin of his fiancée.

Roentgen and the X-ray

In chapter 1, I told of the 1895 discovery of the x-ray, but I did not tell the extent of serendipity involved. German physicist Wilhelm Roentgen (1845–1922) was performing a classic experiment showing how cathode light rays can pass through air for short distances. He used aluminum foil and cardboard to confine the emitted rays, and then, to be sure there were no other sources of illumination, he turned off all lights in the room. Roentgen turned on the cathode ray tube and was astonished to see a fluorescent plate on a workbench across the room emitting a greenish glow, the rays having passed through the materials intended to confine them. He went on to test his rays on a variety of objects, and while doing so he realized that the rays produced an outline of his own hand. He observed, "If my hand is held before the fluorescent screen, the shadows show the bones darkly, with only faint outlines of the surrounding tissues" (Gershen, p. 19). Later, he produced the now-famous roentgenographic film of Frau Roentgen's hand.

Chance played a role in Roentgen's discovery. The fluorescent plate noted to glow was not part of the experiment and only by chance was it in the path of the emissions from the cathode tube. This observation might have been ignored were it not for the subsequent finding that, while holding books and other objects in the path of the rays, the emission could show the bones of his hand. His "prepared mind" recognized the significance of what he had found, and Roentgen became one of the medical princes of Serendip.

Richet and Anaphylaxis

By 1902, thanks to the work of Jenner, Hahnemann, Pasteur, and von Behring, medicine was making steady progress in understanding immunity. About this time, French physiologist Charles Robert Richet (1850–1935) faced a special type of problem. It seems that jellyfish stings from swimming in the waters of the Mediterranean Sea annoyed the royal family of Monaco and their guests. Could Richet help?

If small amounts of a material can produce immunity, could a person be immunized against jellyfish venom? Richet wisely chose to test his theory first on a dog. He injected the dog with a small amount of jellyfish venom. Later, he gave the dog a second injection.

Instead of being protected against the effects of the venom (as Richet hoped), the dog promptly became prostrate and died. Curious that this might be an outcome idiosyncratic to the particular canine, Richet repeated the experiment with other animals, with the same fatal result noted in some instances (3). Although the outcome was unlucky for the experimental animals, Richet's serendipitous discovery allowed the elucidation of extreme sensitivity to allergenic material.

To describe the phenomenon, Richet coined the term "anaphylaxis," from the Greek *an*, meaning "without," and *phylaxis*, meaning "protection." In recognition of his work, Richet was awarded the 1913 Nobel Prize in Physiology or Medicine.

Early in my medical practice days, a neighbor was found collapsed face down in his driveway. His physician, one of my partners at the time, was called urgently to the home. (This was long before we had emergency medical technicians standing by with ambulances.) The only evidence of what was wrong was that, with his last conscious breath, the patient had traced in the dusty driveway the words, "BEE STING." The victim's awareness of anaphylaxis and his scribbled message allowed the physician to administer adrenalin promptly and save his life.

Van den Bergh and His Reagent

In 1913, Dutch chemist A.A. Hijmans van den Bergh (1869–1943) had a bright idea. Paul Ehrlich (1854–1915), who had invented the "magic bullet" arsphenamine, aka Salvarsan (see chapter 1), had also invented a diazo reagent used to test urine to detect liver disease. Van den Bergh asked, quite logically, whether the same reagent could be used as a diagnostic test on serum.

During one of his experiments, van den Bergh neglected to add the alcohol needed to make the reagent and bilirubin dissolve in the test tube. Low and behold, he noted an unexpected pink color in the test tube. He then corrected his error and added the alcohol, only to see the color become a rich violet-red. What van den Bergh had found, quite by accident, was a way to differentiate conjugated ("direct acting") from unconjugated ("indirect acting") bilirubin. A variation of the reagent and the test continues to be used in clinical laboratories today (Weiss, p. 21).

The Medical Student, the Nurse, and Mercurial Diuretics

In 1919, medicine had just three options as diuretics: caffeine, theophylline, and theobromine. None of them was very effective. Mercurials were used clinically at the time, but they were administered only to treat syphilis; one mercurial antisyphilitic used at the time was merbaphen (Novasurol). Mercury's action as a diuretic was discovered by a chance occurrence that involved a clinical error, diligent record keeping, and recognition of the significance of an unanticipated event.

The scene of the clinical error was the Wenckebach Clinic in Vienna. The perpetrator was a third-year medical student named Alfred Vogl, who (writing in 1950) told the story much better than I could. Here is the tale, as quoted by Scholz (4):

"It was on October 7, 1919, that Johanna was admitted to the First Medical University Clinic. She was a patient with congenital syphilis with juvenile tabes. The family physician had been unable to continue her care at home and had asked his friend Dr. Paul Saxl to admit her to his service at the hospital. During rounds, Dr. Saxl asked me, a third-year medical student, to inject 1 cc of salicylate of mercury parenterally every other day. With my Materia Medica still immature, I wrote out an order for a 10 percent solution of mercury salicylate in water. I learned that the compound was insoluble in water. A benefactor appeared in the person of a retired army surgeon with a new mercurial antisyphilitic, Novasurol. Maybe you can use it. On the day of the first Novasurol injection, a tall column indicated that Johanna's urine output had reached 1,200 cc. My report produced a benevolent smile and a rather lengthy but unconvincing discussion of the wavelike rhythm of biologic functions. As it happened, another syphilitic patient was on our ward at that time. After the injection of 2 cc of Novasurol intramuscularly, the patient passed a massive amount of almost colorless urine. Now everyone became genuinely excited. We were repeatedly able to reproduce these miraculous results, causing deluges at will, to the mutual delight of the patients and ourselves. This is the story of how a series of fortunate errors and coincidences resulted in 'a discovery that has completely revolutionized the treatment of congestive heart failure.' The main credit should probably be given to the diligent nurse who, without specific orders, faithfully collected and charted the urine output."

Mercurial diuretics are out of favor today, and in fact, I cannot think of a single clinical use of mercury today. However, during my early years of practice in the 1960s, before furosemide (Lasix) was discovered, we used

injectable meruallide sodium (Mercuhydrin) as a diuretic to treat congestive heart failure and other causes of edema.

Hopps and the Cardiac Pacemaker

Canadian electrical engineer John A. (Jack) Hopps (1919–1998) was working
on the problem of how to restore normal body temperature to patients
suffering hypothermia. One of the methods tested was radio frequency
heating. During his tests, he observed a strange phenomenon. If an animal's
heart stopped beating owing to hypothermia, the heartbeat could be restored
using electrical or mechanical stimulation.

In 1950, following work on artificial cardiac stimulation, Hopps invented
the first cardiac pacemaker. The bulky device was too large for implantation
in the human body and became an "external" pacemaker. Following Hopps'
lead, a Swedish team invented the "internal" pacemaker eight years later.
By that time, no serendipity was required.

Curiosities in Clinical Medicine

Here is a selected group of strange illnesses, several of which illustrate the
various cultural belief systems that health professionals just might encounter. There are scores of curious maladies in clinical medicine, and someday
you may see a patient with one of these diseases or at least consider it a possibility in a differential diagnosis. I think they make interesting reading.

Koro

Unable to describe the ailment better, I will begin with the definition from
my handy *Stedman's Electronic Medical Dictionary*: Koro is "an acute delusional state occurring in Macassars, natives of the Celebes, and other parts
of the East, in which the subject experiences a sensation that his penis is
shriveling or is being drawn into his abdomen. A synonym is shook jong."
There is a variant, found in women, characterized by fear that the breasts
or vagina will atrophy. Magalini and Scrascia (p. 459) go on to explain that
the disappearance of the penis will be followed by death. They report that
the usual treatment is to secure the penis by tying a ribbon around it or
securing it to a wooden box.

Kar describes two cases from East India (5). The author describes one
patient as follows:

"A 41-year-old unmarried, unemployed male from a business family presented with
the complaints of gradual retraction of penis and scrotum into the abdomen. He
had frequent panic attacks, feeling that the end had come. The symptoms had persisted more than 15 years with a waxing and waning course. During exacerbations,
he spent most of his time measuring the penis by a scale and pulling it in order to

bring it out of the abdomen. He tied a string around it and attached it to a hook above to prevent its shrinkage during the night."

The treatment of koro is psychiatric; only 30 percent of patients experience complete recovery.

Morgellon Disease

Morgellon disease is not in *Stedman's Electronic Medical Dictionary*, nor in my current edition of *Dorland's Medical Dictionary*. The disease does appear, however, in the medical literature, and it even has its own foundation, the Morgellons Research Foundation, with 3,492 registered households (6).

According to Savely et al., Morgellons disease is a "mysterious skin disorder" characterized by non-healing skin lesions that extrude fiber-like strands (7). Patients report stinging or crawling sensations and may note "seed-like granules and black speck-like material associated with their skin" (6). The disease may be misdiagnosed as delusional parasitosis. A connection to Lyme disease has been suggested, and some patients respond to antibiotics, suggesting a yet-to-be-identified infectious cause (7).

Jumping Frenchmen of Maine

Sometimes the disease is just called Jumping Frenchmen. *Stedman's* has simplified the name to "jumping disease." The Jumping Frenchmen disease is an extreme startle reaction. In response to an unexpected noise or other stimulus, victims leap, shout, and fling their arms in the air. Who were the jumping Frenchmen? The disease was first noted in lumberjacks of French Canadian descent working in Maine and the Canadian province of Quebec. Since first described in 1878, the disease has been reported in other settings, including Malaysia and Siberia.

Saint-Hilaire et al. explain that the startle response may be attended by echolalia, echopraxia, or forced obedience. They go on to report that in 1885, Georges Gilles de la Tourette (1857–1904) concluded that the Jumping Frenchmen disease was similar to the disease complex we now know as Tourette syndrome (8).

Although a genetic cause has been postulated, Saint-Hilaire et al. conclude that the disease is "not a neurologic disease, but can be explained in psychological terms as operant conditioned behavior" (8).

Kochleffel Syndrome

Another clinical entity missing from my dictionaries is Kochleffel syndrome. Here, I will paraphrase the elegant depiction of the disease by Klein and Kaplinsky (9). In their definitive description of the disease, the authors begin by providing an insightful etymology: In German, *koch* refers to cooking and *loeffel* means "spoon." Thus, a person afflicted with Kochleffel syndrome is someone who stirs up things, as a cook stirs a soup with a ladle. An uncharitable person would call the patient a busybody.

The onset may be abrupt and there are a wide variety of manifestations, with agitated behavior being common. There seems to be disagreement regarding the relative incidence in men and women; men hold that women are affected much more frequently, whereas women hold the opposite view.

Despite the German derivation of the name, the authors report evidence that the disease existed in the time of the early Chinese, Egyptians, and Israelites. The actual origin of the name, despite the apparent connection to known German words, is controversial. Klein and Kaplinsky describe the debate as follows (9):

"The most attractive theory is that the name derives from Dr. Logophilus Acerbus von Kochloeffel (1780–1812), a surgeon who served in Napoleon's army during the invasion of Russia. [He based his theory on the remarkable feats of some army cooks, and] history records that that Dr. Kochloeffel extensively studied this phenomenon and even wrote a fascinating manuscript on the subject, but this was turned down by several journals because the study was not adequately controlled. Dr. Kochloeffel died heartbroken as a result of having made a mountain out of a molehill and having contracted the illness himself."

As a clinician, I might consider the above to be a fanciful hoax except for two important facts: First, Kochleffel syndrome is encountered from time to time; and second, physicians are not immune from the illness.

Kabuki Syndrome

As I began this section of the chapter, I promised myself I would not present a long series of genetic abnormalities, of which there are many—the majority of which most of us will never see. But I chose to include just one—Kabuki syndrome.

In 1980, Kabuki syndrome was described, not surprisingly, in Japan. Patients with this disease have mental retardation plus multiple congenital anomalies, including arched eyebrows and everted lower lateral eyelids, which bring to mind the facial appearance of the make-up of actors in the traditional Japanese theater, *kabuki* (10). More than 100 cases have been reported in Japan (11).

Today, we know that Kabuki syndrome is not limited to Japan. Cases have been reported in South America, and a cluster of patients has been found in a small area in the Netherlands and others have been described in Brazil (11).

ACHOO Syndrome

ACHOO syndrome describes the photic sneeze reflex—the tendency to sneeze when exposed to a bright light. What I find amusing about the disease—which is apparently not uncommon—is the creative origin of the acronym. ACHOO syndrome stands for (and I am not making this up) "autosomal-dominant compelling helio-ophthalmic outburst syndrome." In fact, in 1989, Morris published a paper providing laboratory documentation of ACHOO syndrome, with calculation of the latency of the reflex (12).

Triskaidekaphobia

The fear of the number 13, or anything 13th, may have begun in ancient Babylonian times (ca. 2200 BCE). The Code of Hammurabi lacks 13 in its list. Judas, the 13th person at the Last Supper table, was the disciple who betrayed Christ. The Knights Templar were rounded up and slaughtered on Friday, the 13th, 1314. The 1970 Apollo 13 moon mission experienced an unlucky series of events, and today Formula One Grand Prix racing has no car 13. Whatever the reason(s), triskaidekaphobia is very much part of Western culture.

Ciardi describes the word *triskaidekaphobia* as "a whimsical, British university invention" based on *tris*, "three;" *kai*, "and;" *deca*, "ten;" and *phobia*, "fear" (p. 392). The word is found in *Stedman's Electronic Medical Dictionary*.

Many U.S. hotels are triskaidekaphobic—no 13th floor. Of course, this means that guests on the 14th floor are actually on the 13th floor. Hendrickson reports that Russian Jewish author Sholom Aleichem (1859–1916), whose work became the basis for *Fiddler on the Roof*, had triskaidekaphobia. You will find no page 13 in his manuscripts. He died on May 13, but if you visit his grave in the cemetery in Glendale, New York, you will see that the inscription on his tombstone indicates the date of death as *May 12a, 1916* (Hendrickson, p. 113).

Would you be surprised to learn that I organized the material in this book so that I would have 12 chapters, not 13?

Medical Trivia: Odd Facts That Recall Our History

The following are some seemingly disjointed anecdotes. I include them here because they are just too appealing to leave out of the book. They are listed under three categories: Diseases, Treatments, and Memorable Persons.

Diseases

Heberden, Jenner, Hunter, and Angina Pectoris

The most common cause of death in the U.S. continues to be heart disease, notably arteriosclerotic coronary artery disease, often initially manifest as angina pectoris. The first clarifying description of angina pectoris, and (in fact) the proposed terminology, was in the work of William Heberden

(1710–1801) in 1772 (Gershen, p. 28). *Stedman's Electronic Medical Dictionary* still lists Heberden angina as a synonym for angina pectoris.

It was Edward Jenner (1749–1823), remembered as the man who popularized the smallpox vaccination, who first described a thrombosed coronary artery in a man who died of a heart attack (Gershen, p. 28).

The poignant comment on angina pectoris, however, comes from Scottish surgeon and hero John Hunter (1728–1793). Hunter was a victim of angina pectoris and was well aware of what might precipitate his symptoms. "My life is in the hands of any rascal who chooses to annoy and tease me." Such an event occurred one day at a professional meeting. Upon being contradicted during a public discussion, Hunter suffered chest pain and died (Fortuine, p. 300).

Scurvy

Steele has written a very readable book about medicine in the early American west: *Bleed, Blister, and Purge: A History of Medicine on the American Frontier* (13). Did you know that "a simple vitamin C deficiency called scurvy rivaled cholera as the number-one killer on the frontier"? The disease was of special concern for frontier soldiers because of the tendency of scurvy victims to lose their teeth. A soldier needed his teeth to rip the paper cartridge used to load his rifle. Celery, watercress, and wild onions were used for both prevention and treatment.

Also, Steele describes health care on the 1804–1806 Lewis and Clark expedition to the Northwest. Here we encounter an old favorite, mercury. A mercury-containing purgative called "Thunderclappers" was used to treat various ailments experienced by members of the Corps of Discovery.

Gout

My wife and I recently purchased a La-Z-Boy reclining chair for our vacation home. The origins of our purchase can, with a little imagination, be traced to colonial times. Easy chairs and chairs with padded footstools were initially invented for invalids—persons with acute gout, as well as others with physical handicaps. The first footrests were used to accommodate the painful foot. Originally relegated to the bedchambers, easy chairs and chairs with footrests eventually migrated to the living rooms of even fashionable homes.

Another appliance used by gout sufferers was the crutch, and when the pain and swelling improved, the walking stick—the cane—was used. Because gout was a disease of the affluent (who could afford expensive, uric acid-rich diets), the cane eventually became fashionable. Some medical practitioners carried gold-headed canes, and the object has become linked with physicians. Many medical schools, including our school in Oregon, present a "Gold-Headed Cane" award to the outstanding graduating student.

Syphilis and the Malaria Parasite

Throughout history, we encounter many treatments for syphilis. In 1910, the arsenic-containing arsphenamine (Salvarsan) was marketed as an improvement (read: "less toxic") over mercurial treatment of syphilis. Some three decades later, penicillin would come into general use. In the meantime, the search continued for an effective antisyphilitic. During this time, some observant person noted that sufferers of neurosyphilis seemed to improve if they contracted malaria, with its recurrent high fevers. For a short time, physicians injected syphilitic patients with the malaria parasite in an effort to reproduce the effect (Weiss, p. 12). This treatment is no longer used.

Infectious Mononucleosis

Sometime prior to 1959, Col. Robert J. Hoagland, chief medical officer at the United States Military Academy at West Point, observed that his U.S. Army cadets seemed to develop epidemic infectious mononucleosis a few days after weekend dates. The specific cause seemed to be, to be frank, enthusiastic osculation. "Mono" became known as the "kissing disease." In the end, Hoagland collected a series of "over 500 personally observed patients" (14).

I know that Hoagland's report predates 1959 because in that year, a professor of microbiology told our class of the association of infectious "mono" and kissing, noting that "prevention is just too depressing to contemplate."

Drugs and Other Ingestants

Mandrake

Mandrake (*Mandragora officinalis*) is a plant belonging to the nightshade family (Solanaceae). It is sometimes called Satan's Apple. Mandrake contains tropane alkaloids, including atropine, belladonna, and hyoscyamine. The root is often bifurcated, presenting the appearance of a human figure, which is reported to scream if uprooted. In the words of Shakespeare, "Shrieks like mandrakes, torn out of the earth" (15). The drug has a lengthy history.

For starters, the drug has long been used as an aphrodisiac and to boost fertility. This alleged attribute seems to originate in the Bible, Genesis 30:14–16. Following some family interactions too complicated to recount here, previously barren Rachel consumes mandrake and subsequently becomes pregnant with Joseph.

Another legend holds that Christ was given mandrake-laced vinegar to drink, creating unconsciousness that persisted for three days, until the time of His resurrection.

About 200 BCE, during the Punic Wars between Rome and the Phoenician city of Carthage, the tide of one battle seems to have been turned by mandrake. Soldiers of the besieged city retreated, leaving behind bottles of wine containing mandragora. The Romans promptly occupied the deserted city, celebrated with the wine, fell asleep, and were then overwhelmed by the returning Carthaginians.

A curious ritual attends harvesting of the plant, probably owing to the legend that uprooting can cause death. A cord fixed to the root is tied around the neck of a dog. The dog is then led away until the mandrake is uprooted. The dog then reportedly dies and the mandrake can be safely handled.

Today, European mandrake is used in folk medicine for a variety of intents: as an emetic, laxative, analgesic, sedative, anesthetic, antiepileptic, and aphrodisiac. Its use is considered possibly unsafe even in small doses and certainly unsafe if taken orally in large doses.

Ginseng

Ginseng, as we know it today, comes from the roots of several species of the *Panax* genus of the family Araliaceae. In Asia, ginseng is and has long been highly valued for its medicinal properties. In the U.S., it is vigorously promoted by the health food industry as what *Stedman's* calls a "neutriceutical," intended to augment mental acuity and various bodily functions.

In his diary, George Washington tells of harvesting ginseng, and in the 1780s Daniel Boone was a ginseng trader. Later, large quantities of ginseng were exported from America to Asia, helping to open trade with China (16). Might we consider renewing this exportation as a means of balancing our current trade deficit with Asia?

Quinine

In the 1630s, returnees from the New World brought to Europe a material that could help alleviate intermittent fevers—malaria. The material, quinine, came from the bark of the cinchona tree. Cinchona bark came to be called Jesuits' Bark, probably because the persons who brought the bark to Europe were Jesuit missionaries.

Because of the nickname—Jesuits' Bark—Protestants such as Oliver Cromwell refused to use the cinchona, and only its eventual recognition as the most effective remedy for malaria allowed its 1677 introduction into the *London Pharmacopoeia* (Porter, p. 233).

Bengay

In chapter 5, I described how Lord Lister was incensed to have his name attached to a mouthwash. French pharmacist Jules Bengue had no such misgivings. In 1898, he compounded and marketed a liniment containing menthol and methyl salicylate in a lanolin base. The name of the product is an anglicized version of Bengue's name—Bengay. The product is still available at your favorite pharmacy.

Dopamine Agonists

By now, physicians are well aware of enhanced sexual activity as a peculiar side effect of the dopamine antagonists used to treat Parkinson disease. When first published, the reports conjured images of oversexed octogenarians prowling the halls of nursing homes. Now there is a new side effect to consider.

Dodd et al. have reported 11 parkinsonian patients treated with dopamine agonists at the Mayo Clinic who developed problem gambling. The investigators suggest that pathologic gambling behavior may be a rare side effect of dopamine agonists (17).

Martinis and Dark Chocolate

Well, they are not exactly drugs, but I wanted to share the results of two recent investigations. A study reported in the *British Medical Journal*, which happily will publish such articles, gives a clue as to the extraordinary good health of secret agent 007, James Bond. As you recall, Bond prefers his martinis "shaken, not stirred." The investigators compared shaken and stirred martinis, concluding that "shaken martinis were more effective in deactivating hydrogen peroxide than the stirred variety, and both were more effective than gin or vermouth alone" (18). Deactivating hydrogen peroxide was considered a proxy for health-promoting antioxidant action. The authors make no mention of the venerated vodka martini and hence offer the opportunity for a follow-up study.

Another heart-warming investigation was reported in the *American Journal of Hypertension*. The authors studied 17 healthy non-smoking young adults who consumed dark chocolate or a "sham procedure" described as chewing without chocolate—although how this serves as a placebo control that mimics eating chocolate baffles me.

Nevertheless, the subjects consuming dark chocolate experienced significantly greater brachial artery diameters and arterial flow. Dilated arteries are less responsive to vasomotor stimulation. The study seems to confirm the salutary effects of chocolate, which many of us had already recognized intuitively (19).

Medical Trivia About Some Memorable Persons

Leopold Auenbrugger

Each time you or I percuss a patient's chest, we should honor the contribution of Leopold Auenbrugger (1722–1809), the Viennese physician who in 1754 first advocated percussion of the chest. Auenbrugger should, in turn, honor his father, a wine merchant who taught his son how to measure the amount of wine remaining in a barrel by thumping the wooden sides of the container.

Percival Pott

We recall Percival Pott (1713–1788) for his observation of scrotal cancer in chimney sweeps, not to mention a number of eponymous conditions, including Pott disease and Pott fracture. One day, our hero fell on London Bridge, fracturing his tibia.

Pott refused to go to St. Bartholomew's hospital, where he was an attending physician, declaring that the only capable surgeon in that hospital (himself) was injured. Instead, he splinted his own leg with a board removed from a door on a nearby house and set out for Guy's Hospital.

Benjamin Franklin and Gout

When it came time to draft the Declaration of Independence, Benjamin Franklin (1706–1790) was the senior statesman on the committee of five charged with the writing task. At that time, Franklin was experiencing an attack of the gout and demurred. The job of composing the initial draft was assigned to Thomas Jefferson—who became the lead author of the United States Declaration of Independence.

Charles Darwin

Darwin (1809–1882), the English naturalist who proposed that evolutionary change occurs though natural selection, was supposed to have become a physician. At age 15, young Charles was dispatched by his father to Edinburgh to study medicine, as was the family tradition. Eldredge relates that Darwin developed "... a distaste for the practice of medicine itself. He was especially disturbed by the agonizing screams of surgery patients operated on without anesthesia" (20). Darwin would have been age 15 in the year 1824. Recall that ether anesthesia was not introduced until 1846. Thus, instead of becoming a reluctant physician, Darwin went on to sail on the HMS *Beagle* to the Galapagos Islands and formulate the theoretical tree of life.

Thomas Jefferson and John Adams

Death is both a part of life and a medical event. Here is an intriguing tale of the deaths of two men we all remember. Founding Fathers Jefferson (1743–1826) and John Adams (1735–1826) were signers of the Declaration of Independence, presidents of the United States, and, at various times, close friends and political adversaries. They maintained an ongoing correspondence until their deaths.

What makes the connection between them memorable is the date of their death. Both men, whose lives were entwined with America's independence and with one another, died, each in his home state, on Independence Day, July 4, 1826, exactly 50 years following the birth of the nation they helped found (21).

Mark Twain

Samuel Langhorne Clemens (1835–1910) was an American humorist who took the pen name Mark Twain, recalling his days on a Mississippi River boat. He has been called the first truly American writer. What is remarkable is the coincidence of dates of his birth and death. When Twain was born on November 30, 1835, Halley's Comet came into view. Halley's Comet returned 75 years later when he died on April 21, 1910 (McLain, p. 129).

Abraham Lincoln

Just hours after delivering the Gettysburg Address, Abraham Lincoln (1809–1865) had a sense that he was becoming ill. Upon his return from Pennsylvania to Washington, his disease revealed itself. The diagnosis was varioloid, a mild form of smallpox seen in persons who have some prior resistance. Lincoln did his best to turn a temporary disability to an advantage, using his illness to discourage visits from persons seeking presidential favors. Holzer quotes Abe as saying from his sickbed, "Come in. I have something now that I can give to everybody" (22).

Adolf Hitler

Be aware that the following involves a little conjecture. During World War II, the Allies had an important weapon—penicillin. The Nazis were able to produce only very little of the drug, meaning that German troops' infected wounds were treated with sulfonamides, a much inferior medication for such use.

Adolf Hitler (1889–1945) had a personal physician, Dr. Theodore Morell, who was a champion of polypharmacy. According to Morell's diary, he administered the following drugs to *der Führer*: cocaine eye drops, nux vomica (containing strychnine), atropine, barbitone, belladonna, dihydroxy codeine, amphetamines, testosterone, and (oh yes) vitamins. With this collection of chemicals in his system, it is a wonder that Hitler could get out of bed.

One drug that Morell administered to Hitler was penicillin. One among the several instances recorded was following the 1944 failed assassination attempt. Where did Morell get the penicillin? Wainwright suggests that the drug may have come from the U.S. He writes, "Some of this penicillin appears to have been captured from, or inadvertently supplied by, the Allies, raising the intriguing possibility that Allied penicillin saved Hitler's life" (23).

John, Paul, George, and Ringo: The Beatles

The English rock group that changed the face of popular music in the 1960s went on to sell the most albums of any musical group in history. Their hits included *Lucy in the Sky with Diamonds* and *Sgt. Pepper's Lonely Hearts Club Band*. The profits seem to have done some good for humanity.

The Beatles, with humble beginnings in an undistinguished basement nightclub in Liverpool, signed a contract with EMI Corporation in England. For the musicians, it was not a generous contract. In the initial agreement, the Beatles—all four of them—were to receive one penny for each single recording sold. EMI eventually reaped enormous profits from their success.

In 1971, the EMI Corporation used some of their huge gains to invent the computed tomography (CT) scanner, which may be the Beatles' greatest legacy, as least as far as health care is concerned. And the story explains why, when I first heard of the new magical diagnostic modality in the early 1970s, it was called an EMI scanner.

Medical Writing

Be careful about reading health books. You may die of a misprint.

Mark Twain

I think of myself as both a physician and a writer, and thus my book about medicine would be incomplete without a few tales about medical writing and publication.

As background, we have come a long way in medical publications. At the onset of the Revolutionary War, the body of American medical literature consisted of 20 pamphlets, three reprints, and a single medical book written by an American surgeon named Dr. John Jones (1729–1791) (Bordley and Harvey, p. 71). Jamieson tells an amusing anecdote about our first American medical book author. Jones refused to follow a custom of the times: He would not wear a wig—a fashion accessory popular with urban physicians of the day. His colleagues considered going wigless to be inappropriate behavior for a surgeon and would not consult with him. Eventually, however, Jones' surgical skills became so renowned that the consultants relented. Reluctantly, they welcomed him to the fellowship of physicians, and wigs subsequently lost their popularity (24).

America's first medical journal was the *Medical Repository*, a quarterly publication edited in New York. As new journals go, the *Medical Repository* had a rather long life: 1797–1824. The now-venerated *New England Journal of Medicine* did not come on the scene until 1812; it was originally called the *New England Journal of Medicine and Surgery* (Bordley and Harvey, p. 71).

The first draft of Osler's *The Principles and Practice of Medicine* was written in 1890, but progress was slow. Sir William Osler (1849–1919), like many of us, seemed to be a bit of a procrastinator when it came to writing. His explanation was, "Up to the 40th year a man was fit for better things than textbooks." In 1889, Osler celebrated his 40th birthday and returned to work. To concentrate on the task, he moved from his home to residents' quarters at the Johns Hopkins University Hospital in Baltimore.

All book writers need publishers, and Osler's was Appleton. Osler had some misgivings about his contractual dealings with his publisher and lamented about "selling my brains to the devil" (Bordley and Harvey, p. 153). The book was finally completed in 1892. Osler seems to have recovered from his angst about "selling his brains." He went on to be the sole author of seven editions and co-author of three more before his death in 1919. The book eventually went out of print following publication of the 16th edition in 1947.

In 1988, Dusseau published a book telling the history of the W.B. Saunders Company, long a leader in medical publishing. As a Saunders author at the time, I received a copy of the book. In it are some tidbits of information little known outside medical publishing circles (25). For example, the first edition of *Dorland's Medical Dictionary*, originally called the *American Illustrated Medical Dictionary*, was not written by Dr. Dorland, but by Saunders editor Ryland Green; the book has enjoyed remarkable longevity and is now in its 29th edition.

The *Nelson Textbook of Pediatrics*, first published in 1945 as the *Mitchell-Nelson Textbook of Pediatrics*, is now in its 17th edition. Dusseau tells the story of how the whole Nelson family helped with the first edition. Editing duties were shared with his wife, whom he acknowledges in the preface, and I can personally attest that spousal help in editing is actually quite common. The special contribution to the book came from younger members of the Nelson household: "His daughters Jane and Ann assisted in a hundred useful ways, especially in correlation of corrections and cross-references and in preparation of the detailed index ('Birds, for the, pp. 1–1413' was their work)" (25).

The following is another Saunders story, which a former Saunders editor told me when I first began writing medical books in 1972, and Dusseau later confirmed the salient facts in print (25). In 1947, a young practicing physician visited the Saunders Company offices in Philadelphia. He came from Uniontown, a farming and mining town that is the county seat of Fayette County, Pennsylvania. The editor who told me the story described the doctor, quite uncharitably, as a "baggy-pants country doctor." Those were his words, not mine.

This Western Pennsylvania doctor had an idea for a book, and Saunders was not the first publisher he had approached. No medical editor would take him seriously. After all, Howard F. Conn was not on the faculty at Harvard or the University of Pennsylvania School of Medicine, and he had never published a book before.

As I heard the tale, at Saunders he was passed to newly hired editor, identified in Dusseau's book as Lloyd Potter (25). The book idea was an annually produced, edited reference work that compiled treatment recommendations by experts in various specialties. The book, *Current Therapy*, first published in 1949 and still published annually, had sold more than one million copies at the time of Conn's death in 1982.

Here is a little known fact about Dr. Conn that I learned by reading his obituary in the *Journal of the American Medical Association* (26). During his years in the U.S. Army, Conn achieved some recognition in another way. In his *Willie and Joe* depiction of the American infantry in the European campaign in World War II, cartoonist Bill Mauldin used Conn (then in the U.S. Army) as the model for a concerned Army physician.

An ongoing treasury of scientific satire is the *Journal of Irreproducible Results* (JIR), published from 1955 until 2003. Originally published in Israel, the JIR was later published by Blackwell Scientific Publications from 1990 to 1994. Several anthologies of JIR articles have been compiled, the latest being the *Journal of Irreproducible Results II* (27).

Although the history has been a little erratic, the JIR continues to be active, and you can subscribe at their Web site (28).

Recently published articles include:

Grace D. *All Theories Proven With One Graph*
Sealy K. *Nate P. Leon's Trip to Las Vegas*
Wooldridge M. *Comparing Apples and Oranges: Normalizing Competitive Eating Records Across Food Disciplines*

Speculation: Could It Really Be True?

Sometimes we can be sure about the impact of medical events on the course of history. Examples include the impact of smallpox in the conquest of Aztec Mexico and the role of malaria and yellow fever in the construction of the Panama Canal (see chapter 2). On the other hand, sometimes we look back in time and can only speculate. The following describes some of these instances of conjecture.

Hippocrates and His Writings

The Hippocratic Corpus contains some 70 works, including essays, lectures, books, and 42 case histories. For centuries, young persons recited the Hippocratic Oath upon receiving the degree of Doctor of Medicine. In chapter 7, I cite a number of Hippocratic aphorisms. Yet it is entirely possible that Hippocrates (ca. 460 BCE-370 BCE) actually wrote none of them.

Hippocrates, who advocated the healing power of nature, was renowned as both a healer and teacher. He founded the Hippocratic school of medicine, which, rather than a bricks-and-mortar institution, was a new way of thinking about health care which included inspection, observation, and a code of moral behavior. The Hippocratic school survived in the persons of his students and later followers, who may well have been the actual authors of most or all of the Hippocratic Corpus. Evidence cited is the diversity of writing styles and the diverse subjects covered (29,30). As they are wont to, experts disagree. No matter who is responsible for the organization, syntax, and grammar, the Hippocratic Corpus reflects the observations and philosophy of the "Father of Clinical Medicine."

The Great Plagues, Jesus Christ, and the Rise of Christianity

Did you ever wonder how the teachings of the otherwise-obscure son of a Jewish carpenter became the foundation of one of the world's major religions? Have you ever pondered how, in a world without television or the Internet, the word of Christ came to influence so many in just a few short centuries following his death? Diseases may have played a pivotal role.

Jesus did not write his thoughts, and what we know of his teachings comes largely from the New Testament, notably through the Synoptic Gospels of Matthew, Mark, and Luke. These writings often tell the same tales of Jesus of Nazareth, which include a number of miracles. Cartwright (pp. 22–23) points out that of 20 miracles described by Luke, all but three are related to healing, casting out devils, and restoring the dead to life. In the Bible, Christ called his 12 apostles and "gave them power and authority over all devils, and to cure diseases. And He sent them to preach the kingdom of God, and to heal the sick" (Luke 9:1–2). Early Christianity clearly took on the healer mantle and represented itself as having supernatural healing powers and the potential for occasional medical miracles.

Throughout this time, there were the great plagues. We are not always totally sure which microorganisms were the causes, but the epidemics of the times spread terror across the civilized world. Following the 125 CE plague of Orosius came the plague of Antonius, which lasted from 165 to 180 CE. This epidemic—perhaps smallpox, possibly measles—was brought to Rome by legionnaires returning from conquests in the Levant and North Africa. The plague of Antonius was also called the plague of Galen (120–200 CE), who practiced during this time and wrote of disease manifestations. The plague of Antonius/Galen killed up to 2,000 persons a day in Rome and eventually caused some five million deaths. This was, of course, in a time when the city's population was much less than it is today.

The daily death count in Rome was later exceeded by the plague of Cyprian, named for St. Cyprian, bishop of Carthage. This epidemic lasted from 250 until 266 and killed some 5,000 Romans daily.

Into this fearful world, a religion that spoke of miraculous healing offered hope. Cartwright (p. 23) writes, "Thus, the growth of the Christian Church was stimulated by its specific medical mission in a succession of plagues. . . . Conversions were more numerous at all times of famine, earthquake or pestilences; at the height of the plague of Cyprian, the bishop and his fellow priests in North Africa were baptizing as many as two or three hundred persons a day."

If early Christianity had not been perceived as capable of medical miracles, would it have enjoyed the success we all recognize today? Would it have survived at all?

Plague, Agrarian England, and Sheep

As my wife and I motored through England while on sabbatical in 1990, I was struck by the number of sheep. I came to believe that unless we were in downtown London, we were never out of sight of sheep. Not cornfields, not wheat fields, not many cattle, just sheep. The reason for the ubiquity of sheep can, perhaps, be traced to the Black Death.

As I described in chapter 2, the Black Death was the bubonic plague that spread across Europe in the 14th century, killing up to 75 million persons. Cartwright tells how the Black Death caused a severe labor shortage in the feudal farms of England. The aristocratic landlords were forced to lease their lands to service laborers, called villeins. The word *villein* comes from Latin *villan*, "a landed estate." The velleins were practical individuals, and in contrast to the lords, they recognized that the greatest profit came with the least human labor. Cartwright relates that the vellein "quickly decreased the area of arable and increased his pasture. Even in the strong corn-growing lands of East Anglia, sheep became the farm staple; in the north and west, sheep virtually ousted all other crops. Tudor prosperity depended on wool" (pp. 44–45).

Perhaps if England, and the Western world, had not experienced the Black Death with its attendant labor shortage, my trip through England would have been drives past fields of corn and wheat—not sheep.

Yellow Fever and the Louisiana Purchase

In chapter 2, I told of yellow fever and slavery in America—how the imported African slaves seemed resistant to yellow fever while Native Americans died in large numbers. In addition, the tendency of Africans to be immune to the disease seems to have had some influence on geography. It helped to bring about the Louisiana Purchase in 1803. Here is how it happened.

At the beginning of the 19th century, Napoleon Bonaparte (1769–1821) envisioned a French empire in the New World. He already controlled large pieces of the area—Mexico, some Caribbean islands, and the midsection of America extending from New Orleans to Canada. All that was needed was to exert his dominance.

In 1801, Napoleon's New World power was challenged by a labor uprising on the island of Haiti, then a colony of France. The laborers in Haiti at the time were almost exclusively from Africa, and they had a capable black leader in Toussaint Louverture. Expecting an easy victory, Napoleon dispatched a large military force commanded by his brother-in-law, Gen. Charles Victor Emmanuel Leclerc. Upon arrival in the port of Santo

Domingo, Gen. Leclerc soon realized that he faced an enemy more deadly than the Haitians—yellow fever.

More than 27,000 French soldiers died of yellow fever, while Haitian blacks seemed relatively unaffected by the disease (Oldstone, pp. 49–51). Following the inevitable French defeat, Haiti received its independence, and Napoleon seemed to lose interest in America. In 1803, he sold the Louisiana Territory, land which now makes up about 22 percent of the United States, to President Jefferson for $15 million, or about 3 cents per acre. In the absence of the defeat of the French army by yellow fever in Haiti, would New Orleans still be governed by France, and would the U.S. stretch "from sea to shining sea"?

Hookworm and the U.S. Civil War

The hookworm exists in the small intestine of its host, and from there the eggs are passed to ground with feces. Once in soil, the eggs hatch into infectious larvae. The larvae of the parasite enter the skin of humans when they walk barefoot in areas where feces contaminate the earth. Once in the skin, the hookworm enters the blood, migrates to the lungs, and then enters the gastrointestinal track when phlegm is swallowed. Once in the intestine, hookworm causes a chronic anemia that can be lifelong.

Hookworm long flourished in the warm climate of the Southern U.S., so much so that in the 19th century, up to 40 percent of persons south of the Mason-Dixon line had hookworm (31). In this setting, we turn to the U.S. Civil War of 1861–1865.

In the Civil War, the South may have had the best generals, but the North had superiority of men and materials. Against the odds, the South might have won the Civil War, but it had the handicap of endemic hookworm. The poor, white, rural inhabitants of the South were typically thin, bordering on emaciated, chronically lethargic, and suffered a sallow complexion and the appearance of early aging. They were afflicted with "the germ of laziness" (31). These were the soldiers of Gen. Robert E. Lee's Army of Northern Virginia.

We will never know the full impact of hookworm on the outcome of the war, but from the beginning, the Confederate army had a serious disadvantage in the chronic poor health of a large number of its troops. Robert Penn Warren called them "gaunt, barefoot, whiskery scarecrows" (32). With Gen. Lee in command of a fully healthy army, might the outcome of the Civil War have been different?

References

1. Walpole H. Letter to Horace Mann, January 28, 1754. As quoted in: *Serendipity and the Three Princes*. Remer TG, ed. Norman: University of Oklahoma Press; 1965:6.

2. Roberts RM. *Serendipity: Accidental Discoveries in Science*. New York, NY: Wiley; 1989.
3. Bollet AJ. Medical history in medical terminology. *Res Staff Physician*. 1999;45:60–63.
4. Scholz H. Some historical aspects of the development of cardiovascular drugs. *Z Kardiol*. 2002;91(Suppl 4):34–42.
5. Kar N. Chronic koro-like symptoms—two case reports. *BMC Psychiatry*. 2005;5:34.
6. Morgellons Research Foundation Web site. Available at: http://www.morgellons. org. Accessed May 15, 2007.
7. Savely VR, Leitao MM, Stricker RB. The mystery of Morgellons disease: infection or delusion? *Am J Clin Dermatol*. 2006;7:1–5.
8. Saint-Hilaire MH, Saint-Hilaire JM, Granger L. Jumping Frenchmen of Maine. *Neurology*. 1986;36:1269–1271.
9. Klein HO, Kaplinsky E. The Kochleffel syndrome. Historical review and manifestations of an old-new clinical entity. *Arch Intern Med*. 1983;143:135.
10. Milunsky J, Huang XL. Unmasking Kabuki syndrome: chromosome 8p22–8p23.1 duplication revealed by comparative genomic hybridization and BAC-FISH. *Clin Genet*. 2003;64:509–516.
11. Kabuki Syndrome Network Web site. Available at: http://www.kabukisyndrome. com. Accessed May 14, 2007.
12. Morris HH 3rd. ACHOO syndrome: laboratory findings. *Cleve Clin J Med*. 1989;56:743–744.
13. Steele V. *Bleed, Blister, and Purge: A History of Medicine on the American Frontier*. Missoula, MT: Mountain Press; 2005.
14. Moser RH. How "mono" made the team. *Med Opinion*. 1971; August: 74–77.
15. Shakespeare W. *Romeo and Juliet*. Act 4, scene 3.
16. Slazinski L. History of ginseng. *JAMA*. 1979;242:616.
17. Dodd ML, Klos KJ, Bower JH, Geda YE, Josephs KA, Ahlskog JE. Pathological gambling caused by drugs used to treat Parkinson disease. *Arch Neurol*. 2005;62:1377–1381.
18. Trevithick CC, Chartrand MM, Wahlman J, Rahman F, Hirst M, Trevithick JR. Shaken, not stirred: bioanalytical study of antioxidant activities of martinis. *BMJ*. 1999;319:1600–1602.
19. Vlachopoulos C, Aznaouridis K, Alexopoulos N, Economou, E, Andreadou I, Stefanadis C: Effect of dark chocolate on arterial function in healthy individuals. *Am J Hypertens*. 2005;18:785–791.
20. Eldredge N. *Darwin: Discovering the Tree of Life*. New York, NY: Norton; 2005:22–23.
21. Ellis JJ. *Founding Brothers*. New York, NY: Vintage Books; 2000:248.
22. Holzer H. *The Health of Abraham Lincoln*. MD. February 1983:90–93.
23. Wainwright M. Hitler's penicillin. *Perspect Biol Med*. 2004;47:189–198.
24. Jamieson HC. Men and books: catechism in medical history. *Can Med Assn J*. 1943;48:363.
25. Dusseau JL. *An Informal History of W. B. Saunders Company: On the Occasion of Its Hundredth Anniversary*. Philadelphia, PA: Saunders; 1988.
26. Gunby P. "Country doctor" passes from publishing scene. *JAMA*. 1982; 247:3177.

27. Scherr GH. *Journal of Irreproducible Results II*. New York, NY: Barnes & Noble, 1997; second printing, 2000.
28. *Journal of Irreproducible Results* Web site. Available at: http://www.jir.com. Accessed May 17, 2007.
29. Singer C, Underwood EA. *Short History of Medicine*. New York, NY: Oxford University Press; 1962.
30. Margotta R. *The Story of Medicine*. New York, NY: Golden Press; 1968.
31. Ettling J. *The Germ of Laziness: Rockefeller Philanthropy and Public Health in the New South*. Cambridge, MA: Harvard University Press; 1981.
32. Warren RP. *The Legacy of the Civil War*. New York, NY: Knopf; 1961:57.

11
Misadventures: Myths, Misinformation, Blunders, and Wrongdoing

The spectrum of medical misadventures is wide and multi-faceted. At the benign end of the continuum are the medical **myths**, often charming stories that cause no serious harm, such as the legend—dating to early Roman times—that oysters hold aphrodisiac properties. Next comes medical **misinformation**, bringing somewhat more potential for mischief, such as our long-held belief that estrogen/progestin therapy was quite safe for widespread use to treat menopausal symptoms, a notion that was soberly tempered by a series of articles published as early as 2002 (1). Medical **blunders**, a classic example being amputation of the wrong leg, are misadventures that cause serious harm, generally only to the single patient involved, although (as we will see) there are times in which larger groups suffer consequences. At the far end of the spectrum comes **wrongdoing**, instances of egregious misconduct such as when doctors use their skills against humanity and as a result damage society and the public's confidence in the medical profession.

As I organized my research for this chapter, it was not always crystal clear where to assign specific individuals and actions. Was the 1956 release of thalidomide in Germany a simple lack of information about an unanticipated, but catastrophic, side effect, or was it an unforgivable, preventable blunder? Was Dr. John Harvey Kellogg, remembered today as the man who invented corn flakes, a true believer in the healing powers of cereal grains, a charlatan for his advocacy of electropathy and radium cures, or a deranged opponent of normal sexual activity? Then there is the story of the 1950s spread of acquired immunodeficiency syndrome (AIDS) via polio vaccine in Africa. Is the tale a myth, misinformation, a malicious rumor, or even possibly true? And so, while you may not concur with my categorization of items in each instance, I hope you enjoy the stories that follow.

Medical Myths

Abracadabra

The word *abracadabra*, well known to most children today, came from a mythical Persian sun god (Shipley, p. 3). The word clearly has magical powers: In numerology, its letters add to 365, the number of days in the year. The word is also linked to *Abraxas*, the Gnostic name for the Supreme Being, in whose emanations are 365 spirits.

Because of its supernatural aura, the word, written in a special way, was imbued with healing powers. Written in an inverted pyramid, *abracadabra* was worn around the neck as a talisman to protect against or treat disease or perhaps some troubling life event (Inglis, pp. 79–80). As an example, in the third century CE, Serenus Sammonicus wrote:

> Thou shalt on paper write the spell divine . . .
> Tie this about the neck with flaxen string;
> Might the good 'twill to the patient bring.
> ABRACADABRA
> BRADCDABR
> RACADAB
> ACADA
> CAD
> A

With each descending line in the pyramid, letters disappeared, along with the symptoms or personal problem. Today, the healing myth is all but forgotten, but the mystical properties of the word live on in its use by magicians in their illusions.

Bullet Baby

In 1959, Napolitani reported two unusual cases of wounds of the uterus (2). One of the cases reported involved a U.S. Civil War battlefield incident. In May 1863, a bullet passed through the scrotum of a young soldier, blasting away one of his testicles. In the battle, a young Virginia farm girl was wounded, and somehow testicular material found its way into her pelvis. Nine months later, the young woman gave birth to a baby, while still staunchly claiming her virginity.

In 1982, the story was recounted in the widely read "Dear Abby" newspaper column.

In the original report in the November 7, 1874 issue of *The American Medical Weekly* (1:233–234), surgeon L.G. Capers published an article entitled "Attention gynecologists—notes from the diary of a field and hospital surgeon, C.S.A." He describes how he first attended the injured soldier and then treated a young woman with an abdominal gunshot injury, who delivered a baby boy 278 days later. The surgeon goes on to report that the rifle ball that had wounded both the soldier and the young woman, now a mother, was lodged in the infant boy's scrotum.

Incredible? Yes, it is. What Dr. Napolitani and Dear Abby failed to note is that in a subsequent issue of *The American Medical Weekly*, the editor explained that the article was a humorous invention and that the listed name of the author (Capers) should have been a clue. The so-called bullet baby may be the first of what we now call "urban legends."

As if there had not been enough mythology about this report, the incident has been incorrectly cited as the origin of the exclamation "son of a gun." In fact, the phrase predates the U.S. Civil War and originated with the British Royal Navy. In early times, wives, girlfriends, and prostitutes sailed aboard Royal Navy ships. Pregnancies occurred. Because time in port did not always coincide with childbirth, some babies were born at sea, often in a secluded area between the cannons of the warship. In some instances, the father of the newborn was unknown and the infant was recorded as a "son of a gun."

Penis Captivus

When, during heterosexual intercourse, the vaginal muscles clamp down firmly and the penis cannot be withdrawn regardless of erection status, the condition is called *penis captivus*. The first person to describe a case of *penis captivus* was Egerton Yorrick Davis, writing in 1884 in *The Philadelphia Medical News*. The noteworthy aspect of this otherwise-mundane report is that it was a hoax by none other than Sir William Osler (1849–1919), who served on the editorial board of the journal (3). It seems that Dr. Osler was annoyed by the pedantry of another member of the editorial board, Dr. Theophilus Parvin, Chair of Obstetrics and Diseases of Women and Children at Jefferson Medical College in Philadelphia. Dr. Parvin had authored a presumptuous editorial describing vaginismus and telling of the "grasping" vagina and "captive human penis." But Dr. Parvin's editorial lacked a case to report. Dr. E.Y. Davis (Osler) obligingly supplied the case, albeit a fanciful invention, in a letter to the journal. An excerpt from the letter follows:

"She screamed, he struggled, and they rolled out of bed together and made frantic efforts to get apart, but without success. . . . I applied water, then ice, but ineffectually, and at last sent for chloroform, a few whiffs of which sent the woman to sleep, relaxing the spasm and released the captive penis."

What began as a spoof found its way into the medical literature and was taken seriously for decades. Since the publication of Osler's letter, there have been scattered anecdotal articles and letters debating whether or not *penis captivus* actually occurs. For the record, the clinical entity is not listed in *Stedman's Electronic Medical Dictionary*. However, the literary hoax gives us some insight into the humorous side of Sir William Osler (see chapter 1).

X-ray Eyes

Following the 1895 invention of the x-ray by Wilhelm Roentgen (1845–1922), there was widespread concern for modesty. If the new x-ray could penetrate human tissue, it certainly could allow Peeping Toms using x-ray glasses to see through women's undergarments. But there was soon a commercially available solution, as one firm advertised x-ray-proof knickers (Porter, p. 606). Although we may chuckle at this century-plus-old worry, witness the current concern about airport screening devices.

Tuberculosis and Vampirism

In the late 18th and early 19th century, tuberculosis (TB) came to be associated with vampirism (4). It is not difficult to see how this might happen. Persons with consumption often had pale skin, they might cough blood, and their eyes might be red and swollen. Then when one person in a family was found to have TB, others in the household might lose their health. Although these persons had probably also contracted TB, the suspicion was that the original victim was sucking the life from those nearby.

One way to break the cycle was a method used following the death of the TB patient/suspected vampire. His or her chest was cut open and the heart was burned, thus breaking the vampire cycle.

The Risks of Being Ahead of Your Time

The following story is from Weiss (p. 53); neither he nor I know if it is true, and the tale may truly be another urban legend. It seems that in 1922 in a New England hospital, a bright and daring young doctor was treating a child with suspected bacterial meningitis. He took the adventurous step of performing a lumbar puncture to obtain spinal fluid to aid in the diagnosis. Although this would be considered the standard of care today, in 1922 performing a spinal tap was considered such an "outrageous intrusion that the poor man was stripped of his hospital privileges, then his membership in the medical society, and finally his license" (Weiss, p. 53). The physician lost his ability to practice medicine and spent the rest of his life working on a chicken farm, an outcome that should serve as a stern warning to all who might consider using an unapproved clinical intervention.

Saltpeter as an Antaphrodisiac

Saltpeter is the common name for potassium nitrate, a mineral source of nitrogen and a component of black gunpowder. The word comes from the Latin *sal*, "salt," and *petra*, "rock." Some 55 years ago, when I was in high school, there was a widely circulated myth that saltpeter was an antaphrodisiac that was commonly added to the food served in all-male institutions, which would certainly be a good reason to be in a school where there were both boys and girls.

The myth, of course, is just that—a fiction—and potassium nitrate has no "sexual" effect on humans. Potassium nitrate or saltpeter does, however, have a true, albeit circuitous, medical connection. Georges Gilles de la Tourette (1857–1904) described the syndrome now named for him—the complex that includes facial tics, choreiform movements, and sometimes coprolalia. Tourette practiced in the Salpetriere Hospital in Paris. The hospital took its name from the fact that it had been built on the site of a former gunpowder storehouse (Greshen, p. 36).

Florence Nightingale and Syphilis

There seems to be a persistent rumor that the Lady with the Lamp died of syphilis. A U.K. Web site confirms the existence of the rumor but holds that it is untrue. "No, she died of extreme old age at 90. There is no possibility that she had syphilis." The Web site explains that a priest who was angry about a proposal by the church to honor her started the rumor. In fact, the Web site relates that his rumor succeeded in preventing the honor from being awarded (5).

According to the same Web site, she was almost certainly a virgin, having forsaken marrying an earnest suitor to do God's work instead.

How Sir Alexander Fleming Saved Winston Churchill's Life—Twice

The following is a heartwarming tale, which I have encountered at least three times, once in a pharmaceutical company periodical sent to physicians for leisure reading. The second was the quoted remarks of the 2001 incoming president of the Oregon Medical Association (OMA), printed in the May 4, 2001 issue of the OMA's *The Scribe*. Here is the latter account:

One day a poor Scottish farmer, while trying to make a living for his family, heard a cry for help coming from a nearby bog. He dropped his tools and ran to the bog. There, mired to his waist in the black muck, was a terrified boy, screaming and struggling to free himself. The farmer saved the lad from what could have been a slow and terrifying death.

The next day, a fancy carriage pulled up to the Scotsman's sparse surroundings. An elegantly dressed nobleman introduced himself as the father of the boy the farmer had saved. "I want to repay you for saving my son's life," said the nobleman.

"No, I can't accept payment for what I did," the farmer replied. At that moment, the farmer's own son came to the door of the family hovel. "Is that your son?" the nobleman asked. "Yes," the farmer replied proudly.

"I'll make you a deal. Let me take him and give him a good education." And that he did. In time, the farm lad graduated from St. Mary's Hospital Medical School in London, and went on to become known throughout the world as the noted Sir Alexander Fleming, the discoverer of penicillin.

Years later, the nobleman's son was again near death, stricken with pneumonia. What saved him? Penicillin. The nobleman was Lord Randolph Churchill. His son was Sir Winston Churchill.

My third encounter with the touching narrative was at the Churchill Centre Web page, which asserts that the tale "is certainly fiction." The Web site points out the following (6):

- The ages of Fleming and Churchill at the time alleged do not fit. Alexander Fleming was 7 years younger than Churchill; at the time of the reported near-drowning, Churchill would have been 20 years old.
- Churchill's well-documented life includes no report of nearly drowning in Scotland during childhood.
- When Churchill suffered pneumonia in 1943, he was treated not with penicillin, but with sulfadiazine, which he washed down with brandy.

According to the Churchill Centre, the myth can be traced to a chapter entitled "The Power of Kindness" in a book entitled *Worship Programs for Juniors*, published about 1950. From this humble origin, we see how an engaging, but fanciful, story can be repeated over and over in print, until it (almost) has the ring of truth.

Naming of Rifampin

Rifampin is a bactericidal drug used in the treatment of various infections, including TB. There is an intriguing story surrounding the name of the drug. Haubrich relates that the agent was so named because "the original organic source was found in a wooded area of northern Italy where, at the time, a camera crew was shooting the movie *Rififi*" (p. 194).

Haubrich goes on to attribute the story to an article by Elmer Bendiner printed in the December 15, 1989 issue of *Hospital Practice*. Haubrich remarks that the tale "puts a strain on credulity." On the other hand, Dirckx, one of America's foremost medical etymologists, reviewed the book. In his review, in a paragraph about etymology's unexpected twists, Dirckx seems to substantiate the tale as he comments, "Rifampin is named after the thriller movie *Rififi*" (7).

AIDS and Polio Vaccine

A sad myth holds that human immunodeficiency virus (HIV), the virus that causes AIDS, was spread in Africa by an oral vaccine named CHAT given in the 1950s to approximately a million persons in Rwanda, Urundi, and the Congo. The story holds that the vaccine was grown in the kidney cells of local chimpanzees, some of which were infected with simian immunodeficiency virus (SIV), regarded as similar to HIV. The story achieved wide acceptance after being included in a book by journalist Edward Hooper entitled *The River: A Journey to the Source of HIV and AIDS* (8).

Later studies have shown that, in fact, the vaccine was made from macaque monkey kidney cells, which resist infection with SIV and HIV. Also, a sample of the CHAT vaccine was discovered and found to be free of both viruses (9,10).

Medical Myths on the Internet

There is a staggering amount of medical misinformation on the World Wide Web. I will cover some of these here as medical myths, a descriptor which is admittedly charitable.

Leptospirosis and the Coke Can

The following report has circulated on the Internet (11):

"This incident happened recently in North Texas. We need to be even more careful everywhere. A woman went boating one Sunday, taking with her some cans of Coke which she had put in the refrigerator of the boat. On Monday she was taken into the intensive care unit and on Wednesday she died.

"The autopsy revealed a certain Leptospirose (sic) caused by the can of Coke from which she had drunk, not using a glass. A test showed that the can was infected by dried rat urine and hence the disease Leptospirosis.

"Rat urine contains toxic and deadly substances. It is highly recommended to wash thoroughly the upper part of soda cans before drinking out of them as they have been stocked in warehouses and transported straight to the shops without being cleaned.

"A study at NYCU showed that the tops of soda cans are more contaminated than public toilets, i.e., full of germs and bacteria. So wash them with water before putting them to the mouth to avoid any kind of fatal accident."

The rumor has no basis in truth. Coca-Cola cans are stored in cardboard cases or shrink-wrap, and contamination by rat urine is very unlikely. Rat urine, while unpleasant to ponder, is no more toxic than the urine of other species and does not contain "deadly substances." There is no record of a study comparing the cleanliness of soda cans and public toilets (11). Just to verify, I searched PubMed: No items found.

Dihydrogen Monoxide Dangers

Here is another fear-provoking Internet alert:

Ban Dihydrogen Monoxide!

"Dihydrogen monoxide is colorless, odorless, tasteless, and kills uncounted thousands of people every year. Most of these deaths are caused by accidental inhalation of DHMO, but the dangers of dihydrogen monoxide do not end there.

Prolonged exposure to its solid form causes severe tissue damage. Symptoms of DHMO ingestion can include excessive sweating and urination, and possibly a bloated feeling, nausea, vomiting, and body electrolyte imbalance. For those who have become dependent, DHMO withdrawal means certain death."

As conscientious citizens, you and I should certainly join the campaign to ban DHMO. The city officials of Aliso Viejo, California, considered banning foam cups upon learning that DHMO was used in their production. Then they discovered that dihydrogen monoxide refers to a molecule containing two hydrogen and one oxygen atoms—H_2O, or water (12).

Ogling Breasts Makes Men Live Longer

Not all Internet medical myths are frightening. Here is one that may be considered encouraging, as least for some of us:

"Great news for girl watchers: Ogling over women's breasts is good for a man's health and can add years to his life, medical experts have discovered. According to the *New England Journal of Medicine*, 'Just 10 minutes of staring at the charms of a well-endowed female is roughly equivalent to a 30-minute aerobics workout' declared gerontologist Dr. Karen Weatherby."

The posting goes on to explain that in a controlled trial, those men who looked at busty females had lower blood pressure, slower resting heart rates, and fewer instances of coronary artery disease. It seems that the research method was as follows: The study group of 100 men were instructed to "look at busty females daily," while the 100 men in the control group were instructed not to do so. After an impressively long five years, the study group had lower resting pulse rates, lower blood pressures, and less coronary artery disease. According to Dr. Weatherby, "Sexual excitement gets the heart pumping and improves blood circulation" (13).

There will probably be little disagreement with Dr. Weatherby's last statement, but there is a small problem with the study described: No such research report was ever published in the *New England Journal of Medicine* and PubMed lists no Dr. Karen Weatherby. Could the report all be an imaginative prank?

Antiperspirants, Breast Cancer, and More

An Internet rumor that circulated a few years ago identified antiperspirants and deodorants as the leading cause of breast cancer. The claim is not true, and, in fact, the products are not even under suspicion.

More Internet Myths

Just to finish this section of the chapter, the following are some more inventive Internet medical yarns (14):

- Microwaving food in plastic containers exposes persons to chemicals that can cause cancer.
- Plastic plug-in air fresheners are a serious fire hazard.
- Some name-brand lipsticks contain "cancer-causing" lead. (But not to worry: The Internet site advises that you can test the lipstick for the presence of lead by scratching it with a 24K ring.)
- Procter and Gamble pot-scrubber sponges contain a toxic chemical.
- Tampax Pearl tampons contain "loose fibers" that can cause yeast infection and cervical bleeding.
- Waterproof sunscreen can cause blindness in children.
- And my favorite on this list: The deadly spider *Arachnius gluteus*, aka the "toilet spider," has killed five persons in the Chicago airport. Beware!

Just in case a reader is taking any of these seriously or one of the companies listed is contacting its lawyers, let me state here that all the above are rumors and hoaxes, and all are false.

Misinformation and Misconceptions

The Caduceus Symbol and the Aesculapian Staff

Let us begin this section with a heraldic misapplication. To begin, the Greek god of medicine, Aesculapius, has long been associated with a serpent ever since the day, as the story goes, a snake crawled from the earth and entwined itself on his staff. Aesculapius killed the snake, and then miraculously another snake crawled forth bearing in its mouth an herbal leaf. The second snake placed the leaf on the head of the dead serpent, which subsequently was restored to life. From that moment on, the snake and staff became a symbol of medicine. There is a famous *aesculapion* at Epidaurus in Greece, reported to be the city where Aesculapius was born. At this healing temple, snakes were allowed to crawl on the floors among the patients as they slept at night.

In quite another setting, we find the caduceus of the Greek messenger of the gods, Hermes. The word *caduceus*, in ancient Greek *kerykeion*, is a herald's staff, and hence a symbol of office.

Whereas Aesculapius had one job—caring for the sick and injured—Hermes was assigned many tasks. In addition to his duties as messenger, Hermes was the Greek god of boundaries, commerce, travelers, poets, athletes, and thieves (Gershen, p. 45). He wore winged sandals and a winged cap and carried a herald's staff, with wings and two intertwined snakes.

So how did the caduceus of Hermes come to be confused with the Aesculapian staff of medicine? As examples, the U.S. Army Medical Corps and U.S. Public Health Service insignias include the caduceus. The mix-up might be traced to the fact that alchemists used the caduceus as early as the seventh century to indicate their possession of supernatural ("hermetic") abilities.

Friedlander has written an informative book on the symbol of medicine, tracing the missteps leading to the current confusion (15). Most of the mistakes occurred in the 19th century, and a key error took place in 1871 when the U.S. surgeon general designated the caduceus as the seal of the Marine Hospital Service, destined to become the U.S. Public Health Service in 1889. Gershen (p. 45) states that the change was for aesthetic reasons, whereas Friedlander attributes the adoption of the caduceus by the Marine Hospital Service "because of its relationship with merchant seamen and the maritime industry." Then in 1902, the Army Medical Corps also adopted the caduceus as its symbol, citing the fact that Hermes the messenger at times brought a message of peace (16).

We may arguably say that the current heraldic muddle thus arises with the surgeon general's 1871 decision. Today, there are calls to clarify the symbol and to move to a uniform use of the Aesculapian staff to symbolize medicine. One group calling for the use of the historically correct symbol is the Minnesota Medical Association, whose director of communications is quoted as saying, "If it's got wings on it, it's not really the symbol of medicine; some may find it hard to believe, but it's true. It's something like using the logo for the National Rifle Association when referring to the Audubon Society" (16).

Chilling Evidence and the Common Cold

The common cold occurs very commonly, especially during cold weather. We erudite and evidence-based clinicians know that the common cold is caused by viruses; in fact, some 200 different viruses have been indicted, notably the rhinoviruses. Studies have failed to demonstrate any relationship between acute cooling of the body surface and the common cold, according to a paper from the Cardiff University Common Cold Centre in Wales (17). (Yes, there really is a Common Cold Centre.)

Nevertheless, we get more colds in cool, damp weather than in the warm summer months. Why? Some believe that the lower humidity during the winter months allows viruses to linger about longer. Perhaps cold weather keeps us indoors more and affords more close interpersonal contact. Eccles speculates that "acute cooling of the body surface causes reflex vasoconstriction in the nose and upper airways, and that this vasoconstrictor response may inhibit respiratory defense and cause the onset of common cold symptoms by converting an asymptomatic subclinical viral infection into a symptomatic clinical infection" (17).

Whatever the apparent link between chills and colds, the illness has generated a vast assortment of patent medicines and almost as many home remedies. In 1954, Sir Alexander Fleming, renowned discoverer of penicillin in 1928 (see chapter 1), was quoted as recommending, "A good gulp of hot whiskey at bedtime—it's not very scientific, but it helps" (Strauss, p. 61).

I like the story by Brallier (p. 14) of what happened one day in a restaurant when American actress Billie Burke noticed that the man sitting at a nearby table seemed to have a severe cold. Burke offered her remedy for the cold: "I'll tell you what to do for it. Drink lots of orange juice and take lots of aspirin. When you get to bed, cover yourself with as many blankets as you can find. Sweat the cold out. Believe me, I know what I'm talking about. I'm Billie Burke of Hollywood."

The man graciously acknowledged the advice as he replied, "Thank you. I am Dr. Mayo of the Mayo Clinic."

Patient "Zero"

This tale describes two misconceptions. The story begins in the early 1980s, when we were starting to learn about AIDS. At about this time, a report from the Centers for Disease Control related how a number of cases of the disease could be traced to a "Patient O." Read letter O as in Ohio. By the time this report found its way into the lay press, the index case had become "Patient Zero."

As the story became more elaborate, Patient Zero was identified as a gay Canadian flight attendant who, by virtue of his international travel and apparently heroic sexual activity, spread the virus to sexual partners around the world. These partners pyramided the epidemic by, in turn, sharing the disease with their own sexual contacts.

For a time, the flight attendant (who died of complications of AIDS in 1984) was condemned as the original source of the epidemic among gay men. In fact, AIDS was well established in the U.S. gay community well before the putative Patient Zero began his intercontinental sexual escapades.

Things We Once Thought Were Beneficial

Fashions in medicine change, especially when it comes to therapy. What was a "drug of choice" last year may be considered contraindicated today. It is as if our knowledge has a "sell by" date. If you or I live long enough, we will see some of our favorite remedies fall into disfavor—and then later a few may return to clinical respectability.

In considering shifts in medical thinking, I chose to ignore methods used in past centuries, such as the 18th century practice of treating "griping of the guts" by swallowing lead bullets (Shryock, p. 66). Instead, I focus on changes that have occurred during my lifetime. The following are some medical interventions that not too long ago we believed beneficial but that we now consider unhelpful, or even harmful.

Diethylstilbestrol

From 1938 until 1971, the synthetic estrogen diethylstilbestrol (DES) was prescribed for pregnant women to prevent miscarriage or premature deliveries. The rationale for its use in the beginning was never quite clear and certainly was not evidence-based. In fact, pregnant women taking diethylstilbestrol were never found to have fewer miscarriages or premature births than those who were not treated. Nevertheless, the physician was trying *something*, and what harm could a little extra estrogen cause?

When we count the pregnant women who received the drug and their progeny, both male and female, up to 10 million persons were exposed to the drug before a 1971 FDA bulletin advised against its use in pregnancy because of reports of adenocarcinoma of the vagina in female offspring (18).

We now know that women who received the drug during pregnancy (the "first generation") have an increased risk of breast cancer. Their daughters, the "second generation" or so-called DES daughters, have an increased risk of clear cell adenocarcinoma of the vagina and an even greater risk of breast cancer than their mothers. DES sons may develop non-cancerous epidermal cysts. Current studies suggest that some effects of the drug may occur in the third generation.

Thalidomide

When we think of drugs that first were felt to be helpful but later were learned to be harmful, we think of thalidomide. The drug was first introduced in Germany in 1956 as an extremely safe, non-habit-forming sedative/hypnotic medication. Suicidal patients could consume huge amounts without lethal effect. The drug was considered so safe that it was sold without prescription and often given to children, in which setting thalidomide was sometimes called the "West German baby sitter" (Cartwright, p. 215).

Within a few years, West German physicians were puzzled as they encountered newborn infants with phocomelia—flipper-like appendages caused by a failure of long bones to develop, leaving undeveloped hands and feet attached to the trunk. Eventually, the connection to thalidomide was discovered, and use in pregnant women ceased. The U.S. was spared the debacle because, at the insistence of one concerned and stubborn scientist, the U.S. Food and Drug Administration never approved the use of the drug.

The paradox is that, except for its dangers in pregnant women, thalidomide continues to be a very safe and effective sedative/hypnotic drug. Today, we are finding new uses for the drug, such as in the treatment of relapsed multiple myeloma.

Phenacetin

Until its use was banned in the U.S. in 1983, phenacetin was a widely used non-prescription analgesic, the "P" in APC tablets taken for headache, backache, and many other types of pain. In time, physicians became aware that many persons who used phenacetin-containing drugs developed kidney disease, specifically interstitial nephritis, often with papillary necrosis. I personally encountered several patients with this problem when I practiced in North Carolina in the late 1970s. The incidence of phenacetin-induced nephropathy began to drop after the drug was banned in the U.S., but the disease continues to be a problem in countries where the analgesic compound is still readily available.

Routine Episiotomy During Childbirth

When I was in training in the early 1960s, my obstetric experience was in a Navy hospital, where there were a lot of deliveries, which provided excellent experience for the trainees. Almost all parturients received an episiotomy—

to shorten the second stage of labor—often followed by the use of outlet forceps.

Routine episiotomy is not fashionable in the U.S. anymore. The procedure causes postpartum pain and often difficulty with defecation. Infection can result. In the long term, episiotomy can contribute to dyspareunia.

The procedure is still used at times in instances of shoulder dystocia, breech birth, fetal distress, or forceps delivery. Routine episiotomy, however, is no longer considered ideal medicine in the U.S.

Irradiation of Acne

In the mid-20th century, patients with severe acne vulgaris were sometimes treated with irradiation. We now know that such irradiation can increase the risk of thyroid disease, including cancer. In addition to using it for acne, we irradiated infants found to have a large thymus gland.

Parenthetically, in those days, we the general public were intrigued with x-rays and blissfully unaware of potential hazards. I recall being in a shoe store in about 1950 and having the fit of my new shoes checked by use of an x-ray machine in the store.

Stimulants for the Aged

When I was a young physician in the mid-1960s, a favorite remedy for tired senior citizens was Ritonic, described as a methylphenidate-vitamin-hormone combination. As I recall, it also had a significant alcohol base. This product, a favorite of some older patients at the time, is no longer available. We are, however, seeing an increasing trend toward diagnosing "adult attention deficit hyperactivity disorder" (adult ADHD), with the subsequent recommendation of long-term stimulant use.

Other Interventions Now Out of Favor

Here are a few other therapeutic methods we once used that are currently considered ineffective or possibly harmful and are seldom—if ever—encountered in clinical practice today:

- Use of injectable mercurial diuretics
- Treatment of hypertension using small doses of phenobarbital
- Routine use of intravenous lidocaine to treat patients with acute myocardial infarction
- Monthly injection of vitamin B_{12} for patients complaining of fatigue
- Bed rest and Buck's extension traction for low back strain
- Use of theophylline as a first-line drug for the patient with asthma
- Routine use of estrogen-progesterone combination therapy for minor menopausal symptoms
- Radical mastectomy for small breast tumors

- Autologous bone marrow transplantation for patients with metastatic breast cancer
- Calcium channel blockers as first-line hypertension treatment
- Incision and drainage of pilonidal cysts as first-choice therapy
- Bursting a ganglion of the wrist by striking it with a heavy book
- Routine prescriptions for amphetamine-based appetite suppressants
- Patching corneal abrasions of the eye
- Skull roentgenograms for patients with head trauma
- Antral resection and vagotomy for peptic ulcer disease
- Routine tonsillectomy for recurrent pharyngitis
- Treatment of Herpes zoster infections with protamide injections
- Routine oxygen supplementation for premature infants
- Prolonged bed rest following routine obstetrical delivery
- Prolonged hospitalization with bed rest following acute myocardial infarction

Practices Open to Question

Today we do some things that perhaps we shouldn't. Often the reason given is "for completeness," "to avoid overlooking anything," or frankly to avoid litigation risk. Here are few clinical practices that just might join our Out of Favor list:

- Electronic fetal monitoring of low-risk pregnancies
- Routine use of multivitamin supplements
- Diagnostic imaging of patients with long-term, unchanged migraine headaches
- Antibiotic therapy of bronchitis
- Elective cesarean sections for non-clinical reasons (such as to comply with a school entry deadline)
- Routine complete physical examination of apparently healthy individuals

Things We Once Thought Harmful

The list of things we once thought harmful or ineffective but now consider helpful is not long. Here are the some that come to mind:

Beta-Blockers and Heart Failure

When beta-blocker drugs were first introduced more than three decades ago, we all learned not to give them to patients with heart failure, because the drugs could aggravate the condition. Subsequently, evidence had developed showing that, in appropriate settings, beta-blockers can reduce morbidity and mortality in patients with heart failure.

Watchful Waiting in Otitis Media

The diagnosis for which a child is most likely to receive antibiotics is acute otitis media, accounting for some 15 million prescriptions annually in the U.S. Studies suggest that acute otitis media can be safely managed by use of the "wait-and-see prescription," with the clever acronym WASP. Parents of a child with otitis media receive an antibiotic prescription but are advised not to fill the prescription unless the child is not better or is worse in 48 hours. Such a regimen may become widely accepted as a means to reduce the unnecessary use of antibiotics in children (19).

Back to Sleep

In the past, physicians, if asked at all, recommended that infants sleep in a prone position. This seemed to make sense; if the infant spit up some milk, the prone position would help avoid aspiration. Now, we advise having infants sleep in the supine position—"back to sleep"—which helps to reduce the risk of sudden infant death syndrome (SIDS).

Families in Hospital and Birthing Rooms

Perhaps you recall the days when adult family members would visit hospitalized relatives only during very conscribed hours, and children could not visit at all, lest they carry germs to the patient. Over the past few decades, thinking has changed, and hospitals now are quite liberal with visiting rules. It seems everyone is welcome, including children, and at almost any hour. In fact, with reductions in the nursing staff available, family members often are key members of the care team, whose presence ensures that the patient gets timely service.

A major change has been in the delivery room, where fathers, grandparents, and children once rarely set foot. In a delivery a few years ago, I counted 12 persons in the delivery room, which included the baby's father, the mother of the parturient, and several of her siblings and older children, the medical student, the resident physician, and me. When the baby was born, the number in the room increased to 13.

A Few Others

Some additional interventions that we once shunned but now consider useful are early ambulation following surgery, perioperative use of heparin, and the administration of flu shots to children.

The Jury is Out

There is still controversy about newborn circumcision, routine prostate-specific antigen screening of asymptomatic men, and the long-term risks or value of caffeine use and of vitamin E supplementation.

Medical Blunders

Leaders in American medicine, notably the Institute of Medicine, have recently focused attention on medical errors. There are errors of commission, such as when a patient receives the wrong medicine. Then there are the errors of omission, as in when the patient fails to receive a needed medication. This section of the chapter will mention a few of these but will also describe times when a group of physicians, entire medical specialties, and even society made colossal gaffes, resulting in outcomes that harmed more than one individual, and at times, a great many persons.

John Hunter and the Hunterian Chancre

In chapter 1, I gave some examples of using oneself as a research subject, a practice employed by several of the medical giants described. Scottish surgeon and anatomist John Hunter (1728–1793) engaged in one such experiment. Unfortunately, for Hunter and for the medical science of his time, his self-experimentation was a colossal medical blunder.

As part of his study of gonorrhea in 1767, Hunter inoculated himself with pus from a person with gonorrhea. Unknown to Hunter, the donor was also infected with syphilis. Hunter went on to describe the development of the syphilitic chancre, earning him an eponymous designation of dubious distinction—the Hunterian chancre. In the end, Hunter developed syphilitic aortitis with severe angina, leading to his cardiac death, as described in chapter 10 (Fortuine, p. 300).

Hunter's misadventure also was a setback for medical science. In 1786, he published a paper reporting that gonorrhea and syphilis were caused by the same organism, an erroneous conclusion that endured for a century as a known "fact" in medicine (Major, 1945, p. 45).

Bleeding, Purging, Leeches, and the Standard of Care

More than 2,000 years ago, Alexander the Great of Macedonia (356–323 BCE) died at age 33 of an unknown cause in the palace of Nebuchadrezzar II of Babylon. He may have died as a result of excessive drinking or tainted food, he may have been poisoned, or he may have suffered a relapse of malaria. Whatever the cause, on his deathbed, Alexander remarked, "I die with the help of too many physicians" (Strauss, p. 257).

Today, we can only cringe at the remedies employed by some of our predecessors, methods that, in retrospect, only served to hasten the demise of many patients, even though these practices represented the standard of care at the time. The following are a few examples.

Charles II of England

Charles II (1630–1685), recalled as a generally popular monarch during the time of "Merry Olde England," took the throne following the death of Oliver Cromwell. His final days are described by McKinney (20):

"[Charles II] while shaving fell unconscious in his bedroom. The Royal physicians employed the following treatment. A pint of blood was extracted from his right arm, then eight ounces from the left shoulder, next an emetic, two physics, and an enema consisting of 15 substances. Then his head was shaved and a blister raised on his scalp. To purge the brain a sneezing powder was given; then cowslip powder to strengthen it. Meanwhile more emetics; soothing drinks; and more bleeding; also a plaster of pitch and pigeon dung applied to the royal feet."

All together, over eight days, he received almost 100 drugs. In the words of Sir Andrew Macphail, "In the case report it is recorded that the emetic and the purge worked so mightily well that it was a wonder the patient died" (Strauss, p. 635).

Benjamin Rush and Malaria

By the late 18th century, medical science does not seem to have progressed very much. Dr. Benjamin Rush (1745–1813), "Founding Father of American Medicine," attended the Continental Congress, signed the Declaration of Independence, and later served as professor of medicine at the University of Pennsylvania in Philadelphia. In 1793, Philadelphia suffered a yellow fever epidemic that killed about 1 person in 10 and "raised some doubts about the future of the Quaker City or of other large towns" (Shryock, p. 95). Rush had a heroic regimen for treating the disease. He believed that the fever "stimulated the body" and that the cure must deplete the system. To treat his yellow fever patients, he used calomel (mercurous chloride) purges and profuse bleeding using lancets. Eventually, Rush's copious bloodletting led to a lawsuit, alleging that the physician had killed some patients, a conclusion that we might support today. I will pick up the thread of this case below.

George Washington and the Death of the President

George Washington (1732–1799), first president of the United States and consensus designee as the "Father of His Country," became ill on a cold December day in 1799 with a painful throat and shortness of breath. Three physicians attended him, and Ellis tells us that, "Washington enjoyed the best care that medical science of that time could provide" (p. 268). The best medical science of the day, however, would today be considered colossally harmful.

Washington received the usual purge with calomel and also tartar emetic (antimony potassium tartrate). The boldest therapy, however, was bloodletting, and some five pints of blood were removed from the patient. In the end, Washington died, ironically on the same day that Rush was victorious in the lawsuit over his bloodletting practices (21).

As an interesting aside, on his deathbed, Washington instructed that his body be put into the vault after a delay of two days. He held a fear, not uncommon at the time, that some presumably dead persons—possibly including even Jesus Christ—had been buried before they were really dead (Ellis, p. 269). In fact, the concern over being buried alive explains the use of the word *wake* as part of the funeral process.

President James A. Garfield and the Menace of Too Many Experts

Sometimes I wonder whether power and fame might just be risk factors when it comes to medical care of severe injuries or illness. There is the tendency to involve too many physicians, to take too long with decisions, and—worst of all—to do too much. The death of U.S. President James A. Garfield (1831–1881) is such an example.

On July 2, 1881, less than four months after taking office, Garfield was shot by a political dissident at a Washington, D.C. railroad station. The bullet entered his flank and was not immediately fatal. During the subsequent 11 weeks before his death, physicians searched for the bullet. A porcelain-tipped probe was introduced into the wound, in an effort to snare and remove the bullet. Alexander Graham Bell was consulted; he employed a primitive metal detector in an unsuccessful effort to locate the bullet. In desperation, one physician after another probed the wound with an ungloved finger. Recall that the accepted practice of the time was for the surgeon's hands to be "socially clean" (22).

After 11 weeks of care by some of the most renowned physicians of the day employing the limitless resources available to treat the U.S. president, Garfield died of rampant sepsis, making his the second shortest presidential term in U.S. history, the shortest being that of William Henry Harrison—who died after only one month in office (see chapter 9).

Cocaine Misuse by Physicians

With easy accessibility and often stressful work, physicians are at special risk for misuse of drugs. Others at risk include the affluent and the famous. The history of cocaine misuse illustrates some of the dangers.

Cocaine, an alkaloid derived from the leaves of the coca plant, is a central nervous stimulant that can give the user a sense of increased energy and euphoria. It is also a local anesthetic and is used today for that purpose. In 1884, at the Ophthalmological Congress in Heidelberg, Germany, a live demonstration dramatized the use of cocaine to anesthetize the conjunctiva and cornea (23). In that same year, Dr. Sigmund Freud (1856–1939) published a paper on cocaine—*Über Coca*—which he held to be a "magical substance" that could alleviate fatigue, asthma, headache, depression, and impotence. By the early 1900s, cocaine had achieved wide acceptance in Europe and America and was part of many elixirs and tonics. From 1886 until 1903, cocaine was the signature ingredient in Coca-Cola and is the source of the name of the popular soft drink. In this setting, is there any wonder that well-known persons such as U.S. president Ulysses S. Grant (1822–1885), French actress Sarah Bernhardt (1844–1923), and American inventor Thomas Alva Edison (1847–1931) all used cocaine?

What is disturbing is the number of physicians—both distinguished and unheralded—who fell victim to cocaine. For example, Scottish author and physician Sir Arthur Conan Doyle (1859–1930), best remembered for his Sherlock Holmes stories, used cocaine.

An especially sad tale concerns Dr. William S. Halsted (1852–1922), American surgeon who helped promote the use of protective gloves in surgery (see chapter 10). Soon after the demonstration of cocaine's use in anesthesia, Halsted and some colleagues began to experiment with the drug. At that time, the addictive and destructive potential of the drug was still unknown. Their investigations can be described as inventive and wide-ranging and included treatment of the common cold, use to enhance the experience at the theater (to "add color to the play"), and injections of the drugs into themselves to study its effects (23).

In time, Halsted became addicted to the drug, as did several of his colleagues. With Halsted's stature as the leading surgeon of his generation and professor of surgery at Johns Hopkins University School of Medicine, it is not surprising that his "his addiction was a forbidden topic of open conversation around Johns Hopkins" (24). Eventually, his drug dependence began to affect his work. In May 1886, Halsted entered an institution to treat his addiction, but he continued to suffer relapses and lived a life of "controlled addiction" until his death 36 years later.

Typhoid Mary and Bureaucratic Mismanagement

The tale of Typhoid Mary cannot be considered a public health triumph. The story began with a 1900 outbreak of typhoid fever in New York City. In the best tradition of medical detectives, public health authorities tracked down the source of the infection. The carrier was a poor Irish immigrant girl named Mary Mallon who was working as a cook. As a carrier, she was asymptomatic but could spread the disease to others. Mary was promptly taken into custody, but having committed no crime, was released on the condition that she not seek employment as a food handler. Mary, however, needed work and she returned to her trade as a cook. Another epidemic ensued, and again the outbreak was traced to her.

With no medical remedy for her carrier state, U.S. health authorities designated her a menace to public health, and she was demonized as "Typhoid Mary" (Ciardi, p. 396). Just as John Snow removed the pump handle, health officials removed Mary from society. She was banished for life to Quarantine Island, where she was forced to live alone with her dog for 23 years until her death in 1938 (Porter, p. 424).

Lübeck and the BCG Vaccine

In chapter 2, I told the story of TB. A key breakthrough came with the 1882 discovery by German scientist Robert Koch (1843–1910) of the tubercle bacillus, an advance that set the stage for the development of a preventive vaccine. By the 1920s, a useful immunization had been produced, named Bacille-Calmette-Guérin (BCG) in honor of the scientists who created the vaccine while working at the Institute Pasteur in Paris.

All seemed well until 1929–1930, when 251 babies in Lübeck, Germany, were given the BCG vaccine. Of these infants, 207 developed TB and 72 died of the disease. The immediate conclusion was that the BCG vaccine had reverted to a virulent state. The subsequent investigation and trial brought worldwide publicity.

Eventually, in 1932, the inquiry ended. Findings revealed that the BCG vaccine given to the children had been contaminated with virulent tubercle bacilli. The two physicians responsible for the disastrous mix-up were imprisoned. The incident cast a shadow over the BCG vaccine that would cloud its acceptance for years.

Eleanor Roosevelt and the Treatment of Tuberculosis

America's First Lady from 1933 to 1945, Eleanor Roosevelt (1884–1962) was a Roosevelt through and through. She was the daughter of Elliott and Anna Hall Roosevelt, the niece of Theodore Roosevelt, and the wife of Franklin Delano Roosevelt. By about 1960, she developed manifestations of TB. Instead of prescribing the antituberculous antibiotics available at the time (Streptomycin was discovered in the 1940s), her physicians prescribed corticosteroids, which would exacerbate rather than help her TB.

Why did this therapeutic misjudgment occur? Let me suggest a hypothesis: Cortisone was discovered by American chemist Edward C. Kendall (1886–1972) in the late 1940s, earning Kendall and two colleagues the 1950 Noble Prize in Physiology or Medicine. The drug's commercial production and distribution by Merck followed some time later. By 1960, we were approaching the end of our honeymoon with the new wonder drug, still enchanted with its benefits and just beginning to appreciate its problematic traits. I suspect that the ailing First Lady found that the cortisone therapy increased her vitality and enhanced her mood; the exacerbation of her TB would come later.

Freedom for Psychotic Patients in the U.S.

Most medical missteps involve a single individual or a small group of persons, but one modern misadventure involved an entire nation—the U.S.

This error in judgment was the decision about four decades ago to release chronically ill patients in psychiatric hospitals and to do so abruptly and without much planning about how to care for them outside the walls of an institution.

In 1954, chlorpromazine (Thorazine) was approved for psychiatric use in the U.S. The antipsychotic agent seemed a wonder drug, analogous to what the antibiotics had proven to be. This new medication to control schizophrenia came into widespread use during the 1960s—the era of the civil rights movement, the sexual revolution, women's liberation, and a general distrust of government and institutions. In those days, we eschewed experts and espoused self-reliance. Releasing the many "imprisoned" persons in psychiatric hospitals was quite consistent with the mood of the times. Tens of thousands of medicated schizophrenic men and women were discharged to unprepared local families and communities. Today, we have huge populations living on the streets and in our prisons. Surprise.

The Tired Trainee, the Serotonin Syndrome, and Resident Work Hour Rules

In March 1984 in a New York hospital, a tired resident physician who had been on duty for 18 hours ordered the administration of meperidine (Demerol) to a young woman who had arrived at the hospital having earlier taken the monoamine oxidase (MAO) inhibitor phenelzine (Nardil). The patient developed serotonin syndrome, a medication-induced condition characterized by excessive serotonergic stimulation of the central nervous system and peripheral receptors. The patient died following respiratory arrest. Her father (a journalist and attorney) sued, citing the unusual claim that his daughter's death was the result of care rendered by fatigued and unsupervised physician trainees. A jury found no criminal fault but agreed with the plaintiff's depiction of the care received.

The patient's name was Libby Zion, and following her death a New York law was passed in 1989 that limits the number of resident work hours. In 2003, the Accreditation Council for Graduate Medical Education followed suit and set work hour rules, which include a maximum workweek of 80 hours per week, averaged over four weeks.

In this case, a medical blunder was sadly lethal for the patient but resulted in rule changes that promise to improve the quality of care in U.S. teaching hospitals and to enhance the quality of life of medical resident trainees.

Care Gone Wrong: Frauds, Quacks, and Rogues

In this section of the chapter, we move from medical blunders—more or less honest mistakes—to wrongdoing. If, as in the words of Robert Louis

Stevenson (see chapter 8), the physician "is the flower (such as it is) of our civilization," then medical misdeeds by physicians must be considered especially shameful.

I believe that medical wrongdoing spans a spectrum. At one end of the scale are dubious practices and deception, instances in which a kind-hearted reader might argue that the perpetrators truly believed that they were doing the right thing. At the other extreme are examples of misconduct that even the most open-minded person must condemn. For example, as I will tell below, one physician became a pirate who plundered coastal towns in South America.

John Hunter and the Giant

Whereas John Hunter's self-inoculation with syphilis in 1767 was a blunder, in another instance he seems to have strayed beyond the bounds of civilized behavior. Hunter (1728–1793) was both surgeon and anatomist, and he was an avid collector of odd specimens. To obtain dissection material, he sometimes employed body snatchers—also called resurrectionists—to dig up graves of the recently departed.

One highly desirable specimen was an Irish giant named Charles Byrne, whose remains Hunter craved for anatomical study. For Hunter, there was only one small problem, and that was that Byrne was not dead. The giant did, however, have advanced TB and Hunter presumed that he would soon die. In an effort to secure the corpse immediately following death, Hunter hired thugs to stalk Byrne as he walked the streets of London.

Byrne soon became aware of the plot to steal his body upon death and arranged for his remains to be spirited to the Irish Sea and sunk in fathoms of water, denying Hunter his coveted anatomic specimens. Hunter, ever the cunning man, outsmarted the giant. The doctor bribed the undertaker, who stole the body for Hunter as the burial party slept while on their journey to the coast. Stones were substituted for the body in the casket, which was ceremoniously dispatched at sea.

Moore suggests that Hunter's sinister behavior may have inspired Robert Louis Stevenson, whose depiction of the doctor's home in the *Strange Case of Dr. Jekyll and Mr. Hyde* is modeled after Hunter's London residence, which was built with a formal entrance for social visitors at the front and a rear entrance for delivery of cadavers (25).

Franz Mesmer and the Magnetic Institute

Viennese physician Franz Anton Mesmer (1734–1815) developed what he considered a novel and effective medical intervention; his index case was a woman with recurrent seizures who responded to therapy with magnets placed on her body. Mesmer postulated a vital force called "animal magnetism" and began to employ his theory in practice. After condemnation by reputable Viennese physicians, Mesmer moved to Paris, where he found a more receptive setting.

In the City of Lights, Mesmer established the Magnetic Institute, aided by Louis XVI and Marie Antoinette. His specific treatment methods included group sessions involving iron rods dipped in magnetized water, hypnotism, and astrology. Mesmer targeted the affluent as patients, one of whom was the Marquis de La Fayette (1757–1834), later to become General Lafayette in the American Revolution.

In 1784, a now-suspicious Louis XVI appointed a commission to investigate animal magnetism. Their conclusion was that Mesmer's treatment had no scientific basis. His support dwindled, and Mesmer departed Paris in 1785 (Porter, pp. 285–286). The last 20 years of his life produced nothing worthy of historical note, but Mesmer did leave a legacy—the word *mesmerize*, meaning to spellbind or hypnotize.

Lydia Pinkham and Her Vegetable Compound

There really was a Lydia Pinkham, born Lydia Estes in 1819 in Massachusetts, whose early life included nursing, midwifery, and teaching, as well as an ironic advocacy for temperance. At age 24, Lydia married a wealthy real estate investor named Isaac Pinkham. When the Pinkham fortune suffered a reversal in 1875, Lydia concocted an herbal tonic, which she branded with her own image on the bottle label and began to sell as a remedy for cramps and various other gynecologic problems, including uterine prolapse. In fact, in the spirit of gender ecumenism, an early label claimed effectiveness for "all weaknesses of the generative organs of either sex."

The tonic was called "Lydia E. Pinkham's Vegetable Compound," and it contained black cohosh, unicorn root, cramp bark, gentian, and iron, all in an impressive 40-proof alcohol base. For those unfamiliar with distilled spirits, a 40-proof elixir is 20 percent alcohol; the vodka you buy at your local liquor store is typically 80 proof, or 40 percent alcohol by volume. Lydia's tonic provided quite a kick, not bad for a concoction devised by a temperance advocate.

Lydia E. Pinkham's Vegetable Compound was one of many patent medicines affected by the Pure Food and Drug Act of 1906. Following the enactment of the law, the tonic's label was revised several times, changes once described as by the American Medical Association (AMA) as, "Lydia Pinkham had changed her dress again." By 1939, the label made the following bland and profoundly unhelpful claim: Lydia E. Pinkham's Vegetable Compound is "recommended as a vegetable tonic in conditions for which this preparation is adapted" (26).

Robert Koch and His Secret Remedy

In 1882, German physician Robert Koch (1843–1910) discovered the tubercle bacillus that causes TB. His breakthrough was attributable, in part, to a novel culture technique. To create the successful culture medium, Koch combined blood with the agar his wife used to make jam.

If Koch had stopped there, his life story would be untainted, but he not only tried to take shortcuts in science, he also entered the perilous world of commerce. In 1890, Koch told the world that he had developed a cure for TB. The world cheered the historic discovery. His remedy was called "tuberculin," although Koch carefully avoided disclosing the nature of the compound.

In an age long before evidence-based medicine and with Koch coasting on his fame as the discoverer of the tubercle bacillus, the new secret remedy was given to thousands of TB patients without benefit of adequate testing or controls. Eventually, tuberculin proved to be, at best, valueless and sometimes harmful as a remedy for pulmonary TB. In 1891, Koch disclosed that the mystery drug was simply a glycerin preparation of tubercle bacilli. Porter reports that Koch fled to Egypt with a new young wife and also perhaps with the funds received from a pharmaceutical company to whom he had sold his remedy before its nature was exposed (p. 441).

Ironically, Koch's tuberculin was noted to cause swelling and redness at the injection site. Eventually, this reaction became the basis for the tuberculin skin test we use today.

The Cereal Doctors

Sylvester Graham

There were three "cereal doctors," all of whose names are familiar to us today because of products they developed. In their days, they had some peculiar ideas. The first was Sylvester Graham (1794–1851), an American Presbyterian minister, self-styled physician, and advocate of both vegetarianism and temperance. His followers were called Grahamites. Graham deplored chemical additives in food and his contribution to today's diet comes from Graham bread, invented in 1829 and made from chemical-free whole-wheat flour. One of Graham's passions was to curb sexual lust, and to this end he recommended celibacy for men until age 30 and subsequently a maximum of one sexual encounter per month. His bland Graham bread was part of the ascetic regimen. Today's grocery store graham crackers were named for him, but they differ from the original formula by containing honey or molasses and—sometimes—refined flour.

John H. Kellogg

Next came Dr. John Harvey Kellogg (1852–1943). While superintendent of the Battle Creek Sanitarium at Battle Creek, Michigan, John and his brother Will serendipitously "cooked up" the idea that evolved into corn flakes in the early 1890s. The sanitarium was on a tight budget, and one day when the brothers had allowed some cooked wheat to become stale, they decided to produce some potentially usable long sheets of dough by forcing the material through rollers. Instead of sheets of dough, they got flakes. Sensing possibilities, they toasted the flakes and served them to patients, who seemed to like the taste and texture. They filed a patent for the product in 1894, and the American cereal industry was born.

If only Dr. John Kellogg had stopped there and built on his cereal success. However, he had other keen interests. In the sanitarium, he practiced mechanotherapy, electropathy, and radium cures. He was an advocate of a healthy bowel and employed an enema machine that could deliver 15 gallons of water to the bowel in only a few seconds. He decried masturbation, advocating circumcision "without administering an anesthetic" for small boys, and the application of carbolic acid to the clitoris of girls (27).

It seems that Kellogg opposed not only masturbation, but heterosexual activity as well, and that he never had sexual intercourse with his wife. The seven Kellogg children were all adopted.

Those interested in seeing a humorous adaptation of Kellogg's quirky methods should view the 1994 motion picture *The Road to Wellville*, based on the 1993 novel of the same name by American author T.C. Boyle.

C.W. Post

After Kellogg came C.W. Post (1854–1914), a former Kellogg employee who founded the rival Postum Cereal Company in 1895. Their first breakfast cereal, Grape-Nuts, was marketed two years later. Then came Post Toasties, his brand of corn flakes.

Post, like his predecessors, had some odd beliefs about nutrition. One of his dictums was, "When a man has approaching symptoms of appendicitis, the attack can be voided by discontinuing all food except Grape-Nuts" (28). Ironically, Post committed suicide in 1914 shortly after surgical removal of his appendix.

Classic Quackery

The quack has been called "the Physician of the Fools" (Strauss, p. 482). Garrison observes, "The tendency to consult quacks is analogous to the physician's liability to be deluded by wild-cat investments" (p. 782). The word *quack* comes from the early Dutch word *quacksalver*, meaning one who quacks—like a duck—about his salves. Train (p. 50) reports that the word arose during the 14th century bubonic plague as charlatans sought to victimize terrified people hoping for a miracle.

Whispering Physicians

Early quacks were the "whispering physicians" of Germany, who claimed knowledge of health-restoring herbs and who, for a fee, would quietly describe the promised remedy, speaking softly into the patient's ear.

James Graham

Inglis (p. 120) describes a classic quack, James Graham (1745–1794), a self-proclaimed doctor who never actually completed his medical studies. Graham's contribution to the tales of quackery was the Temple of Health, featuring the Celestial Bed. The London home of the Temple, opened in 1780, featured Aesculapian symbols and scantily clothed young female attendants. The Celestial Bed, itself a massive 4 yards long and 3 yards wide, was supported by 40 glass pillars. As couples lay on the bed, they listened to music and breathed scented air and periodically were treated to jolts of electricity that allegedly created a magnetic field. Those who could afford to spend a night in the Celestial Bed were assured that they would not suffer sexual dysfunction or sterility and that they would be "blessed with progeny."

John R. Brinkley

Despite medical training at several medical schools of dubious quality, John R. Brinkley (1885–1942) was licensed to practice medicine. Brinkley is remembered today for his goat gland surgery, which began in 1918. For a fee of merely $750, Brinkley held that he could cure male impotence and infertility by surgical implantation of goat glands. By 1928, Brinkley had become a target of the AMA, owing to his use of advertising to solicit patients. In 1930, his Kansas state medical license was revoked, ending his career as the "goat gland doctor."

But Brinkley was not going to quit without a fight. In an effort to gain the political power needed to appoint sympathetic members to the state board of medical examiners—members who might restore his license—Brinkley ran for governor of Kansas three times—in 1930, 1932, and 1934. He did not win any of these elections.

Albert Abrams

A once-respected physician who had served as vice president of the California Medical Society, Albert Abrams (1863–1924) introduced the Electronic Reactions of Abrams (ERA), also called Radionics, in 1916. Abrams held that the key to diagnosis and therapy of illness is electrons and that every disease has its own electronic vibratory rate, which can be measured by one of his remarkable devices.

How remarkable were his instruments? Using the Dynomizer, a drop of blood or even a sample of the patient's handwriting would be all that was needed to diagnose what was wrong. Following the ERA diagnosis, the patient could then be treated with vibratory waves created by the Oscillo-clast. Abrams shared his machines and offered training, for a fee, and at the height of his success in 1921, some 3,500 clinicians were using ERA in their practices.

After a faulty diagnosis in 1923, Abrams, like Brinkley, attracted the attention of the AMA. In the investigation and controversy that followed, one interesting event involved the submission of a blood sample to a clinician using ERA diagnosis; the unfortunate patient was diagnosed as having the unlikely quartet of cancer, diabetes mellitus, syphilis, and malaria. The source of the blood sample was a rooster—that presumably enjoyed good health.

Before the legal wrangling could be concluded, Abrams died of pneumonia. Shortly following his death, the AMA explored the technology inside an ERA device. What they found was nothing more than a rat's nest of wires, buzzers, and lights.

Iridology

Do you think quackery has disappeared in the 21st century? Think again. A case in point is iridology, aka iris diagnosis, which holds that there is an area on the iris of the eye that corresponds to each area of the body. Thus, examination of the pigment spots of the iris can allow the diagnosis and localization of disease. Iridologists claim that they can diagnosis a number of "imbalances" that respond to herbs, vitamins, minerals, and supplements. These health-restoring products can be conveniently purchased in their offices—or through multi-level distributors.

To check on the current status of iridology, I googled the words "iridology practitioners." At the top of the list was the Web site for the International Iridology Practitioners Association, announcing their annual symposium this year in Las Vegas, Nevada.

Fake Cancer Cures

It seems to me that there must be very few actions in medicine more hateful than preying on the hopes of those with advanced cancer. Yet history is full of such tales. One of them concerns Laetrile.

Laetrile

Laetrile is the proprietary name for amygdalin, a derivative of bitter almonds, apricot pits, and some other nuts and fruits. The drug attained popularity beginning in the 1970s as a treatment for cancer, allegedly acting by selectively killing cancer cells. As reputable physicians learned more about the drug, problems surfaced.

First of all, Laetrile turned out to be not as safe as originally claimed. In the body, the drug is metabolized to yield benzaldehyde and hydrogen cyanide. Serious side effects were reported, and a few cyanide poisoning deaths occurred.

Perhaps Laetrile's side effects might have been acceptable if the drug was highly effective, but it was not. A multi-center U.S. trial failed to show any therapeutic benefit at all. The drug is no longer used by reputable American physicians but is still available to desperate cancer patients at a few clinics in Mexico.

Other Bogus Cancer Cures

The list of fake and questionable cancer cures includes a number of creative interventions. Here are some of them:

- A mistletoe extract named Iscador was popularized as a cancer remedy in the 1920s. It seems that the time the plant is picked is crucial, necessitating the optimum alignment of the moon, sun, and planets. Perhaps a problem with picking times is the reason why no benefit to cancer patients has ever been substantiated.
- Beginning in 1949, thousands of cancer patients were treated with krebiozen, originally described as derived from an odd source—the blood of Argentinean horses that had been injected with *Actinomyces bovis*, the bacterial cause of actinomycosis in cattle. Subsequently, krebiozen was discovered by the U.S. Food and Drug Administration to be nothing more than the chemical compound creatine.
- Macrobiotics, suggesting *the way to a big* (long?) *life*, holds that the key to preventing and "relieving" cancer and other diseases is to balance the *yin* and *yang* foods. Practitioners also employ ancestral diagnosis, spiritual diagnosis, and astrological diagnosis.
- Proponents of shark cartilage treatment hold that it contains a protein that blocks the proliferation of new blood vessels needed to allow the growth of cancer.
- The notion that oxygen deficiency causes cancer is the basis of hyperoxygenation therapy. Cancer patients are treated with ozone, hydrogen peroxide, or similar products.
- American chemist Linus Pauling (1901–1994), the only person to win two unshared Nobel Prizes, popularized the theory that high-dose vitamin C can treat cancer. Following years of consuming megadoses of the vitamin, his wife Ava and then Pauling himself died of cancer (in 1981 and 1994, respectively).
- One of the most inventive fake cancer cures is psychic surgery, whose practitioners claim to remove diseased organs without creating a surgical incision in the skin. Chiefly practiced in the Philippines and Brazil, psychic surgery is not limited to cancer patients. Psychic surgeons claim to be able to cure diabetes, headache, and backache. Skeptics hold that psychic surgery is based on sleight-of-hand techniques and the gullibility of suffering patients.

Thomas Dover, the Pirate Doctor

Among the rogues, the pirate doctor is Thomas Dover (1662–1742). Before becoming a pirate, Dover accumulated impressive medical credentials. He attended both Cambridge and Oxford and then apprenticed with Thomas Sydenham (1624–1689). During one of the many conflicts between England and Spain, Dover abandoned his general practice, outfitted a warship, hired a pirate crew, and set sail for the west coast of South America. There he and his men did what buccaneers do—they sacked Spanish-held cities in Chile and Ecuador. At the end of three years, Dover and his men returned to England, bringing home great wealth from the New World.

Not content to retire and enjoy a life of affluent leisure, Dover returned to medical practice. He went on to develop a sedative combination of opium, lactose, and ipecac known as Dover's Powder, which is not listed in my current reference books.

Joseph Guillotin

French physician Joseph Guillotin (1738–1814) was deputy to the National Assembly during the French Revolution of 1789–1799. At that time, the wealthy landlords and other members of the nobility were busily being executed, often in clumsy ways, notably by beheading with a sword, which required both dexterity and strength to be accomplished cleanly. To increase efficiency and to reduce suffering, Guillotin devised an apparatus that could swiftly decapitate a revolutionary. The date of the first execution by guillotine was April 25, 1792. Eventually, the device would be used to end the lives of Louis XVI and Marie Antoinette in 1793. Dr. Guillotin will forever be remembered as the doctor who created an instrument of death.

Compromising Trust in Physicians and Scientists

I cannot end this chapter on medical misadventures without mentioning what I consider two of the most egregious acts of physicians and scientists—inappropriate human experimentation and falsification of scientific data.

Inappropriate Human Experimentation

Physicians who perform unethical human experiments betray their oath. Here, I will briefly describe two examples: the Tuskegee Syphilis Study and events that occurred in Nazi concentration camps during World War II.

Beginning in 1932, in Tuskegee, Alabama, 399 impoverished, poorly educated, and syphilitic African Americans and 201 non-infected controls were enrolled in a study of the natural history and therapy of the disease, formally entitled the Public Health Syphilis Study. By the late 1940s, penicillin had become both widely used and recognized as accepted therapy of syphilis. The study subjects, however, were denied both penicillin and information about its availability and effectiveness. The study continued in this manner until terminated in 1972, following an exposé in the *Washington Star* and a subsequent report in the *New York Times*. Later, the Tuskegee study was the basis for the 1992 stage play entitled *Miss Evers' Boys* and a subsequent 1997 made-for-television motion picture.

During the Second World War, the Nazis set out to exterminate the Jewish population and other "undesirables." Less well known is that the killing began a few years earlier, in 1939, when Hitler ordered the "euthanasia" of state hospital inmates who were mentally disabled or terminally ill—"eradicating life unworthy of life" (29). After the beginning of the war, methods of killing large numbers of persons were adapted for use in Nazi concentration camps.

In these camps, Nazi physicians descended one step further, using inmates as human subjects in some terrible experiments to study the effects of freezing, drowning, gangrene, mustard gas, and petrol injections. Some inmates were simply murdered to provide cadavers for dissection (Porter, p. 649). Following the end of the war, surviving Nazi physicians were bought to trial and punished, but no amount of retribution could erase society's memory of these evil physicians and the atrocities they committed in the name of medical science.

Scientific Fraud

If inappropriate human experimentation can shake our faith in the humanity of physicians, scientific fraud can undermine our trust in research investigators. A recent example concerned a paper on stem cell research (*Stem Cells* 2004;22:950–961). The paper evoked "serious concerns," including the statement that an involved professor had "fabricated at least some of his stem cell research." In a discussion of the issues published in the involved journal, Civin writes, "The currency of science is the peer-reviewed and peer-accepted manuscript that is 'backed by a gold standard' of scientific integrity and scrupulous honesty. Anything that tarnishes this 'gold standard' threatens to devalue the worth of scientific currency. Ultimately, society itself suffers because scientific advancement prepares the way for societal progress" (30).

References

1. Rossouw JE, Anderson GL, Prentice RL, et al., for the Writing Group for the Women's Health Initiative Investigators. Risks and benefits of estrogen plus progestin in healthy postmenopausal women: principal results from the Women's Health Initiative randomized control trial. *JAMA*. 2002;288:321–333.
2. Napolitani FD. Two unusual cases of gunshot wounds of the uterus. *N Y State J Med*. 1959;59:491–493.
3. Altaffer LF 3rd. Penis captivus and the mischievous Sir William Osler. *South Med J*. 1983;76:637–641.
4. Citro JA. *Passing Strange: True Tales of New England Haunting and Horrors*. Boston, MA: Houghton Mifflin; 1997.

5. Frequently Asked Questions (about Florence Nightingale). Available at: http://Florence-nightingale-avenging-angel.co.uk.faq.htm. Accessed May 20, 2007.
6. Fleming saved him from drowning: "Sir Alexander Fleming Twice Saved Churchill's Life." The Churchill Centre. Available at: http://www.winstonchurchill.org/i4a/pages/index.cfm?pageid=102. Accessed May 20, 2007.
7. Dirckx JH. Review of: Haubrich: medical meanings: a glossary of word origins. *JAMA*. 1997;278:688–689.
8. Hooper E. *The River: A Journey to the Source of HIV and AIDS*. Boston, MA: Little, Brown; 1999.
9. Blancou P, Vartanian JP, Christopherson C, et al. Polio vaccine samples not linked to AIDS. *Nature*. 2001;410:1045–1046.
10. Berry N, Jenkins A, Martin J, et al. Mitochondrial DNA and retroviral RNA analyses of archival oral polio vaccine (OPV CHAT) materials: evidence of macaque nuclear sequences confirms substrate identity. *Vaccine*. 2005;23: 1639–1648.
11. Woman catches leptospirosis from unwashed Coke can—Netlore Archive. Available at: http://urbanlegends.about.com/library/bl_coke_can_leptospirose. htm. Accessed May 20, 2007.
12. Safety warning: dihydrogen monoxide (DHMO)—Netlore Archive. Available at: http://urbanlegends.about.com/library/bl_ban_dhmo.htm. Accessed May 20, 2007.
13. Ogling breasts makes men live longer. Available at: http://urbanlegends.about. com/library/weekly/aa072600a.htm. Accessed May 20, 2007.
14. Current Netlore: Health/Medical, Internet hoaxes, email rumors and urban legends. Available at: http://urbanlegends.about.com/library/blxhealth2.htm. Accessed May 20, 2007.
15. Friedlander WJ. *The Golden Wand of Medicine: A History of the Caduceus in Medicine*. New York, NY: Greenwood Press; 1992.
16. Caduceus confusion: group wants right symbol. *Am Med News*. 1994; Nov 7:16.
17. Eccles R. Acute cooling of the body surface and the common cold. *Rhinology*. 2002;40:109–114.
18. Herbst AL, Ulfelder H, Poskanzer DC. Adenocarcinoma of the vagina: association of maternal stilbestrol therapy with tumor appearance in young women. *N Engl J Med*. 1971;284:878–881.
19. Spiro DM, Tay KY, Arnold DH, Dziura JD, Baker MD, Shapiro ED. Wait-and-see prescription for the treatment of acute otitis media: a randomized controlled trial. *JAMA*. 2006;296:1235–1241.
20. McKinney J. *Early Medieval Medicine*. Baltimore, MD: Johns Hopkins Press; 1937.
21. Morens DM. Death of a president. *N Engl J Med*. 1999;341:1845–1849.
22. Bollet AJ. Wounded presidents: 1981 almost repeats the events of 1881. *Med Times*. 1981;109:19–23.
23. Nunn DB. Dr. Halsted's addiction. *Johns Hopkins Adv Stud Med*. 2006;6:106–108.
24. Olch PD. William S. Halsted and local anesthesia: contributions and complications. *Anesthesiology*. 1975;42:479–486.
25. Moore W. *The Knife Man: The Extraordinary Life and Times of John Hunter, Father of Modern Surgery*. New York, NY: Broadway Books, 2005.

26. Lydia Pinkham's new dress. *Time*. January 2, 1939. Available at: http://www.time. com/time/magazine/article/0,9171,760553,00.html. Accessed May 22, 2007.
27. Kellogg JH. *Treatment for Self-Abuse and Its Effects, Plain Fact for Old and Young*. Burlington, IA: F. Segner & Co; 1888.
28. Karlen A. A capsule history of nostrums. *Phys World*. 1974;11:59–66.
29. Bryant MS. *Confronting the "Good Death:" Nazi Euthanasia on Trial, 1945–1953*. Boulder: University of Colorado Press, 2005.
30. Civin CI. Cloned photomicrographs, not cloned cells. *Stem Cells*. 2005: Dec 28; Epub ahead of print. Available at: http://www.ncbi.nlm.nih.gov/entrez/query.fcgi? db=pubmed&cmd=Retrieve&dopt=AbstractPlus&list_uids=16382036&itool= iconfft&query_hl=1&itool=pubmed_DocSum. Accessed May 20, 2007.

12
Now and Future Practice

In the past 11 chapters, we have visited some heroes, diseases, and treatments that are part of the heritage of the healing professions, we have discussed some of the language of medicine and some thoughts of our most erudite predecessors, and we have examined some instances of clinical practice, including a few times when what happened was not what we today would have wished. I hope that the 231 pages that we have traveled together so far have convinced you of the rich and (usually) honorable traditions of medicine. The tales are sometimes epic, at times tragic, sporadically triumphant, and occasionally lamentable. This last chapter suggests some ways that you, as a health professional or informed consumer, will now—I hope—learn more about medicine's history and lore.

Recommended Reading

When seeking to learn more about anything, and especially what has happened in the past, books are a great place to start. Of course, you may be thinking, "The computer and the Internet are replacing books." Perhaps this will be true some day; certainly e-mail has replaced handwritten letters as a means of personal correspondence. We should all grieve this loss of civility and of what should become of valuable historical records. Imagine what would have happened if the correspondence of Thomas Jefferson and John and Abigail Adams had been via e-mail, read by the recipients and then deleted forever.

As I wrote this book, I did a great deal of research on computer, as well as in books and scientific journals. The computer can provide fast facts: The Internet was invaluable in allowing me to tell dates of birth and death for persons mentioned in the various chapters; it permitted me to do a lot of important fact-checking. However, the Internet could seldom provide the context of facts presented and the linguistic richness of books. The World Wide Web lacks the thoughtful, often lyrical prose found in the best-written books. Also, with a book or article, I know who to blame if facts are wrong; the Internet is much more impersonal.

And so with that introduction, let us look at selected books that may help you learn more.

Osler's Recommendations

Sometime around 1904, Sir William Osler (1849–1919) collected a number of his addresses "delivered at sundry times and diverse places in the course of a busy life." The book's title is *Aequanimitas with Other Addresses to Medical Students, Nurses and Practitioners of Medicine.* On the last (and curiously unnumbered) page of the book, the one item in the book (other than the preface) that is not a record of an address is Osler's recommendations for a "Bedside Library for Medical Students" (Osler, last page):

"A liberal education may be had at a very slight cost of time and money. Well filled though the day be with appointed tasks, to make the best possible use of your one or of your ten talents, rest not satisfied with this professional training, but try to get the education, if not of a scholar, at least of a gentleman. Before going to sleep read for half an hour, and in the morning have a book open on the dressing table. You will be surprised to find how much can be accomplished in the course of a year. I have put down a list of ten books which you may make close friends. There are many others; studied carefully in your student days, these will help in the inner education of which I speak.

    I. Old and New Testament
   II. Shakespeare
  III. Montaigne
  IV. Plutarch's *Lives*
   V. Marcus Aurelius
  VI. Epictetus
 VII. *Religio Medici*
VIII. *Don Quixote de la Mancha*
  IX. Ralph Waldo Emerson
   X. Oliver Wendell Holmes—Breakfast Table Series"

I have actually read some of Osler's recommended books. I recall that in high school, a Spanish teacher and mentor excused me from class for a few days so that I could read Cervantes' *Don Quixote de la Mancha.* I do my best to see a Shakespearean play each year. I have read bits and pieces of several of the other authors and works recommended.

Taylor's Recommendations

Inspired by Osler, I hereby humbly offer a list of 12 recommended books. Yes, my list has two more books than Osler's, but it is, after all, a century later. I chose these books from the Bibliography that follows this chapter, and hence some are reference works. My recommended books all have to do with medical history, and some incidentally present epistemology and moral values in a medical context. A few of these read like mystery novels, some are inspirational, and all tell facts we physicians should know. Here is the list, with some annotations:

- Ackerknecht EH. *History and Geography of the Most Important Diseases.* New York, NY: Hafner; 1972. This is a manageable book (210 pages, including the index) that traces the demographics of the major communicable diseases, plus deficiency diseases, diseases of unknown origin, and more.
- Bordley J. *Two Centuries of American Medicine, 1776–1976.* Philadelphia, PA: Saunders; 1976. A reference work of 844 pages, *Two Centuries* traces medical history from the founding of the United States until its bicentennial in 1976, the year of the book's publication.
- Cartwright FF. *Disease and History: The Influence of Disease in Shaping the Great Events of History.* New York, NY: Crowell; 1972. This readable book does just what the subtitle promises. It traces the influence of disease—such as typhus, syphilis, and the Black Death—on events in world history.
- Dirckx JH. *The Language of Medicine: Its Evolution, Structure, and Dynamics.* 2nd ed. New York, NY: Praeger; 1983. Perhaps I am assuming an elitist posture, but of all the medical word origin books available, I prefer this one for its scholarly approach. Dirckx discusses medical words in the context of our classical traditions, historical curiosities, modern coinages, slang, and jargon.
- Durham RH. *Encyclopedia of Medical Syndromes.* New York, NY: Harper and Brothers; 1960. If you want to know about the "stiff-man" syndrome, egg-white syndrome, or bullous malignant erythema multiforme syndrome (Stevens-Johnson syndrome), this is the place to look. Virtually all the popular and lesser-known eponymous diseases are here.
- Garrison FH. *History of Medicine.* 4th ed. Philadelphia, PA: Saunders; 1929. Garrison's is the "Bible" of medical history books. In my opinion, it is still unequaled in scholarship. Would you believe that as a young physician, I read this 996-page book cover to cover? My well-worn copy bears the underlining to support this claim.
- Martí-Ibáñez F. *A Prelude to Medical History.* New York, NY: MD Publications, 1961. The foreword to the book begins, "I am a lover of the spoken word. No violin rendition, no piano recital, no symphonic concert can transport me as does a well-turned lecture." The book is a collection of the author's lectures to medical students of the New York Medical College, Flower and Fifth Avenue hospitals. The astute reader will note that I have begun and ended my book with quotes from Martí-Ibáñez.
- Osler W. *Aequanimitas with Other Addresses to Medical Students, Nurses and Practitioners of Medicine.* 3rd ed. Philadelphia, PA: Blakiston; 1932. Mentioned above in reference to the "Bedside Library for Medical Students," Osler's collection of addresses retains its inspirational qualities a century after its initial publication in 1904.

- Porter R. *The Greatest Benefit to Mankind.* New York, NY: Norton; 1997. With the subtitle *A Medical History of Humanity*, this book is an ambitious, but comprehensible, story of the human side of medicine.
- Sebastian A. *The Dictionary of the History of Medicine.* New York, NY: Parthenon; 1999. Do not attempt to read this book for pleasure. Sebastian's *Dictionary* is an epic reference work weighing almost six pounds. In it you can find discussions of the Ebers papyrus, liver extract, and the Royal Society of London.
- Strauss MB. *Familiar Medical Quotations.* Boston, MA: Little, Brown; 1968. Strauss has assembled the most useful of all collections of medical quotations, not surprising in that, in the preface, the author describes his long-term attention to the task: "Just when I began collecting medical quotations remains a mystery. The yellowed scraps of paper suggest a minimum of twenty-five years ago." Every physician who writes or who delivers lectures should have this book in his or her library.
- Weiss AB. *Medical Odysseys: The Different and Sometimes Unexpected Pathways to 20th Century Medical Discoveries.* New Brunswick, NJ: Rutgers University Press; 1991. This book, telling stories of the often convoluted and occasionally unexpected routes to discovery, could be enjoyable bedtime reading.

Landmarks in Medical History

A good friend once told me, "There are two kinds of people in the world—those who travel and those who don't." Sometimes it's good to get out of the office and travel. When traveling in your own country or abroad, take some time to visit medical landmarks—historical sites and museums that recall medical history. Sometimes they are a little hard to find; the typical tourist is probably not likely to seek out the Semmelweis Museum in Budapest or the Museum of Questionable Medical Devices at the Science Museum in St. Paul, Minnesota. However, visiting the site of an important medical event or a collection of medical artifacts can become the highlight of a trip.

Here is a list of some suggested medical landmarks to visit. Some merit an afternoon excursion if you happen to be visiting a city; others, such as the Greek Island of Kos, represent worthwhile travel destinations.

Europe and Greece

Kos

From the balcony of our hotel in Kos, we could see Turkey across the waters of the Karpathian Sea. My wife and I visited Kos in 2002 with a group of fellow physicians. Kos, of course, was the home of Hippocrates (ca. 460–377 BCE), and here we visited the two chief medical history attractions of the island.

The first, in a quiet city square, is the Plane tree—or at least a descendent of the original tree—under whose branches Hippocrates taught his pupils. The other awe-inspiring medical site is the Aesculapion, the temple of healing built in the fourth century BCE. Here, the physicians in our group recited in unison the Oath of Hippocrates on a bright, sunny morning in October.

Epidaurus

On the northeast coast of the Peloponnesus lies the ancient city of Epidaurus. Here was built the Aesculapion, a center of healing well known throughout Greece (mentioned in chapter 11). Sick persons came to spend the night in the sleeping hall, the *enkoimitiria*, where during the night Aesculapius might help them find their way back to health. The pilgrims to the Aesculapion brought riches to the city and allowed the construction of the nearby amphitheater, famous for its remarkable acoustics.

Baths of Caracalla

Some may hold that the Baths of Caracalla in Rome are not truly a medical attraction, but I include them to highlight that public health measures— including providing clean water and other advances in sanitation—were the chief medical contributions of the ancient Romans. Built in the early third century CE during the reign of Emperor Caracalla, the baths are worth a visit during the day or perhaps on a summer evening when the ruins are the backdrop for the *Teatro del Opera di Roma*.

Anatomy Theater in Padua

The oldest anatomy theater in the world is in Padua, Italy, and it was here that Andreas Vesalius (1514–1564) conducted his anatomic dissections. The remarkably well-preserved auditorium is part of the University of Padua. Among the other noteworthy persons who taught at the University were Copernicus, Galileo, and Giovanni Battista Morgagni. You will probably need a guide to find this well-preserved architectural treasure among the many halls and rooms of the university.

The Hunterian Museum in London

In 1783, our own ubiquitous John Hunter, recalled for making surgery a scientific discipline as well as for his syphilitic misadventure and his eventually fatal temper, began what is now the Hunterian Collection of the Royal

College of Surgeons in London. The collection holds thousands of specimens, including 3,500 of Hunter's original preparations, such as a specimen showing his successful ligation of the femoral artery for popliteal aneurysm.

Semmelweis Museum in Budapest

The home of Ignaz Semmelweis (1818–1865) in Budapest, Hungary, is now the site of a small museum showing artifacts from his life and a selection of other antique medical items.

The Handleless Pump in London

We recall that, in 1854, John Snow (1813–1858) helped stop a cholera epidemic in the Broad Street neighborhood of London (see chapter 1). A short walk from Leicester Square in Soho is Broadwick Street; in 1936, the suffix "wick" was added to the name of historic Broad Street—in my opinion, a sad distortion of historical nomenclature. You will not find a formal museum. What is there may be even better: There is a handleless pump, a commemorative plaque, and the John Snow Pub, with some framed memorabilia of Snow's work. Ironically, Snow did not drink alcohol, and yet the only building honoring his memory is a tavern.

Pasteur Museum in Paris

Nestled in the Pasteur Institute in Paris is the Pasteur Museum, opened in 1936. Here you will find mementos of the life and work of French microbiologist Louis Pasteur (1822–1895), whose work and name give us *pasteurization*. You can view the apartment where Pasteur and his wife lived, and you can visit Pasteur's tomb.

Asia and the Middle East

National Museum of Medical Science History of the Islamic Republic of Iran

This museum, opened just a few years ago in Tehran, presents Iran's historical contributions to medical science. The exhibits draw on an inventory of "more than 3,000 objects, tools, pictures, documents, and books related to medical sciences" (1).

Traditional Chinese Medical College

Although most medical schools in the People's Republic of China lean toward an allopathic, "Western" approach to medicine, there are still some traditional medical colleges in China. In 1980, I visited one such medical college and hospital in Beijing, where I witnessed acupuncture, moxibustion, cupping using short pieces of bamboo, and cauterization of enlarged tonsils in children. (The children, wide awake during the procedure, felt no pain. The tonsils have no nerve fibers that conduct pain.) Shanghai, for example, has the Museum of Medical History of Shanghai College of Traditional Chinese Medicine. If the Chinese city you are visiting has a traditional medical college, a tour of the facilities will be memorable.

The United States

Ether Dome

You can tour the Ether Dome at the Bullfinch Building of Massachusetts General Hospital in Boston, Massachusetts, where William T.G. Morton (1819–1868) conducted his now-famous demonstration of ether anesthesia (see chapter 1).

National Library of Medicine

In Bethesda, Maryland, is the National Library of Medicine. It is simply the world's largest medical library. Visitors are welcome and tours are available. For information, visit their Web site (2).

Museum of Questionable Medical Devices

In St. Paul, Minnesota, is the Museum of Questionable Medical Devices at the Science Museum of Minnesota. Here you can see the psychograph, the vibrometer, and the foot-operated breast enlarger.

Other Medical History Museums and Sites

I could make this a very long list; there are hundreds of museums and sites around the world with medical significance. In Europe, consider visiting the Uppsala (Sweden) Museum of Medical History, where you can view the world's first obstetrical forceps. Consider also the Berlin Medical Historical Museum in Germany and the Western Australia Medical Museum in Perth. Consult your guidebook and use the Internet to find these places as you travel.

In the U.S, there is the Dittrick Medical History Center of Case Western Reserve University in Cleveland, Ohio. If you are visiting Indianapolis, Indiana, spend some time in the Indiana Medical History Museum. In Frederick, Maryland, you can visit the National Museum of Civil War Medicine. Countless American cites and towns have sites of medical interest; a good reference source is Lipp's book *Medical Landmarks USA: A Travel Guide to Historic Sites, Architectural Gems, Remarkable Museums and Libraries, and Other Places of Health-Related Interest* (3).

Thoughts Upon (Almost) Completing the Manuscript for This Book

This section is a personal indulgence, and it is risky for two reasons. The first is that I am stating—in print—some of my opinions, and a few of them have prognostic overtones, thus exposing myself to scorn if I am proven wrong in the future. The second risk is that opinions can be challenged, although such questioning should be considered an invitation for dialogue.

After reading the readable books and consulting the reference sources listed in the Bibliography, after spending hundreds of hours searching PubMed and other Internet sites, and after following the trail of scores of clues that might explain curious tales, I have formulated some thoughts. Here they are:

1. The Age of Self-Experimentation Is Over

John Hunter, Louis Pasteur, Pierre Curie, William T.G. Morton, Joseph Goldberger, and others all used themselves as experimental subjects. Wilhelm Roentgen took the first x-ray film—of his wife's hand. Jonas Salk injected his whole family, as well as himself, with his new polio vaccine. The days of heroically putting one's health, and that of one's family, at risk are gone and should not be lamented.

Today, human experimentation is performed under tight control. We in academic medicine sometimes grumble about the administrative hurdles placed in our path by institutional review boards and government agencies, but they help to ensure that episodes such as the Tuskegee Syphilis Study will not be repeated.

2. In the Future, Most Discoveries That Change the Course of Medical History Will Be Made by Teams

As I worked on this book and looked for the name of the single pioneering scientist responsible for breakthroughs in the mapping of the human genome, the control of the hemorrhagic fevers, and the new advances in treating acquired immunodeficiency syndrome (AIDS), I found lists of team members, but no Pasteur, Ehrlich, or Salk. In future books of medical tales, the great advances will be attributed to institutes, consortia, and teams, with the names of the individual scientists often ignored. Happily, Nobel Prizes still recognize individual scientists and physicians.

The ascendance of research teams and the twilight of the lone investigator do not mean that the single, stubborn innovator has vanished entirely from the scene. Furthermore, the traditional bias against novel advances that challenge current dogma is alive and well. More than 20 years ago,

Portland, Oregon otolaryngologist John Epley, MD developed what he believed was an effective and non-invasive treatment for benign paroxysmal positional vertigo. It was a simple maneuver involving moving the body to reposition particles in the inner ear canals. No surgery and no medication were needed. The technique came to be called the Epley maneuver and eventually involved a rotating, computer-controlled chair used to standardize movement of the patient. A 2006 investigative report in the Portland newspaper, *The Oregonian*, tells the reaction of Epley's colleagues: "Inexplicably, they rejected him, heaved accusations that threatened his license to practice medicine." Today, however, the Epley chair is gaining acceptance, has garnered several million dollars in federal grants, and may be on its way to a medical clinic near you (4).

3. Chance Still Favors the Prepared Mind

Pasteur's words still ring true, but many discoveries are made differently today than in the past. Instead of happy accidents and Eureka moments, investigators today may study hundreds of compounds hoping that one will prove clinically useful (and commercially successful). Nevertheless, Dr. John Eng must have had an "Aha" experience when he first realized that a drug for diabetes, now marketed as exenatide (Byetta), might possibly be derived from the venom of the Gila monster. Because he was a Veteran's Administration (VA) employee and because the VA was not interested in seeking a patent, Eng paid for the patent himself and subsequently licensed the patent to a pharmaceutical company (5). Eng shows that there is still a place in medical science for the persistent, intuitive entrepreneur.

4. Medicine's Linguistic Treasury Continues to Grow

The language of medicine is far from dead. Every year, we create new medical words, phases, syndromes, abbreviations, acronyms, euphemisms, jargon, and slang. During my lifetime, and perhaps yours, we have had the following additions to *medicalese*: AIDS, human immunodeficiency virus, prion, erectile dysfunction (well known to all who view television today), nutraceutical, telemedicine, and eHealth. In prior chapters, I described jersey finger, runner's knee, Legionnaires disease, Fred Astaire legs, and the Salk vaccine. A few paragraphs ago, I told of the Epley maneuver; this technique is not in my current edition of *Stedman's Electronic Medical Dictionary* but probably will be at some point in the future. We have developed a host of new abbreviations, acronyms, and slang expressions: WASP (wait-and-see prescription), PET (positron emission tomography), SARS (severe acute respiratory syndrome), and EMR (electronic medical record). We also have learned the meanings of commonly used abbreviations such as NSAID (non-steroidal anti-inflammatory drug) and some that are more specialized, such as UVAL (ultraviolet argon laser). Medicine can take less pride in the creation of squash (brain), fascinoma (an interesting and unexpected clinical finding), and positive gown sign (painting a somewhat graphic image of a patient who exits the hospital with neither permission nor street clothes).

How rapidly is medicine's vocabulary growing? The first edition of what we know as *Dorland's Medical Dictionary* was published in 1890, with the title *American Illustrated Medical Dictionary* (see chapter 10); it had 770 pages. (For temporal orientation, Osler's text *The Principles and Practice of Medicine* was first published in 1892.) By 2000, when the 29th edition of *Dorland's* was published, the book had ballooned to 2,088 pages describing 121,000 items. In 2003, the 30th edition discussed 125,000 items in 2,200 pages. In four short years, we added 4,000 new medical words, phrases, and abbreviations.

Yes, staying current in medicine today involves knowing not only new tests, drugs, and procedures, but new medical words and their permutations.

5. A Medical Scholar Can Do a Lot of Research Quickly on the Internet; Not Everything Found There Is Accurate

For example, I told above about Dr. John Eng paying for the patent for what is now the drug exenatide with his own money. Although the Internet has several sites telling about Eng and his discovery, the only source I could find telling about his personal payment for the patent was http://www. mendosa.com/monster.htm (5). This Web site is entitled Mendosa.com, with the subtitle: Your On-Line Diabetes Resource. The author is David Mendosa. I like Mendosa's story about Dr. Eng and his patent. Is the story accurate? Because Mendosa's piece provides no reference citations, I am not quite sure. In online research for this book, I tended to trust Web sites that are sponsored by government agencies, specialty organizations, and peer-reviewed publications. With appropriate skepticism, I pondered facts presented by Web sites maintained by advocacy groups, such as organizations concerned with single diseases (e.g., Morgellon disease), and I skipped by Web sites whose URL (uniform resource locator) contains words such as Aquarius, underground, and celestial.

6. Some of the Heroes Described in This Book Lived and Died During My Lifetime

These include Alexander Fleming (died in 1955), Abraham Flexner (died in 1959), and Jonas Salk (died in 1995). I wish that I had met these men. While I was in medical school, I heard a lecture by famed pediatrician and book editor Waldo E. Nelson. While in private practice in upstate New York, I met cardiologist Paul Dudley White when he spoke at a county medical society meeting; he struck me as a kind, humble man. If you get the chance to hear or meet a medical giant—or a rising star—be sure to take advantage of the opportunity.

7. The Best Days of Medical Advances Are Ahead of Us

By no means have all the colorful tales of medicine been lived and written. Every scientific advance has the potential to set the stage for several more. I won't try to be Nostradamus and predict specific events in the future, but during the lifetimes of today's young physicians, we can hope to see effective vaccines for the infectious diseases to which we are currently vulnerable (e.g., AIDS), some means to prevent cancers of various types, and interventions to help patients avoid chronic diseases such as diabetes mellitus and hypertension.

8. Until Medical Schools and Residencies Offer Courses in Medical History, Culture, and Linguistics, There Will Be a Need for Books Like This

From time to time, I mention an event in medical history to a medical student or resident. Every month, when I teach a headache seminar for third-year students, I tell the story of ergot and St. Anthony's fire. I describe how Lewis Carroll might have visualized some characters in *Alice's Adventures in Wonderland* as part of a migraine aura visual distortion. I note too many blank stares. Only a few synaptic connections.

   Fortunately, when I attended Temple Medical School long ago, we had some excellent lectures in medical history. I recall the image of Joseph Auenbrugger (1722–1809), inventor of percussion as a diagnostic maneuver, tapping on wine barrels filled to various levels. Could anyone in our class forget the story of how René Laennec (1781–1826) invented the stethoscope in 1816? Embarrassed to place his ear directly on the chest of a young woman he was examining, Laennec rolled several sheets of paper to make a tube that could carry sound from her chest to his ear. I wonder how many of today's young physicians learn these stories. I suspect not many. Until we senior physicians once again assume responsibility for passing on the oral history of our discipline, books like this will be needed.

9. Some Medical Truths Are Best Learned From Patients, Not From Books

I will share one example, humorously encapsulated by Woody Allen: "Eighty percent of life is showing up." I remember one day that—counter to all logic—I drove 18 miles over snowy roads to make a very routine hospital visit to an elderly patient. As I entered the room, she smiled and said, "I knew you would come." That day I felt especially proud to be a physician, and the snowy drive home didn't seem as long as the trip to the hospital.

A less happy lesson was learned in my very first year in practice. My patient, an older man, quite overweight and severely diabetic, was dying. He and his wife lived in a trailer about 40 minutes from our medical group's office. One day, not unexpectedly, his wife awoke to find that her husband had died at home during the night. As was local practice at the time, a physician was needed to go to the home to pronounce him dead. Our group had a designated "house call" physician each day, and this was not my day. My office schedule was full. What should I do? I kept seeing my scheduled patients and dispatched the "house call" doctor to my patient's home. He pronounced the patient dead, doing the job that needed to be done.

The next time I saw the widow, she began to weep. "Why didn't you come when he died? He was your patient." If there are ever times when persons remember every detail of what happens, it is at times of major life events; death is one of these.

You really can't learn lessons such as these from books.

10. Physicians Enjoy the Trust and Privilege We Do Today Because of the Dedication and Sacrifice of Generation of Healers That Have Gone Before Us—Only a Few of Whom Are Described in These Pages

Medical students and young physicians often do not understand this simple truth and seem to assume that the faith and respect that patients accord them is something that they somehow merit.

With few exceptions, our patients do trust us. For the experienced physician, the trust comes from past actions, but it comes also from patients' subconscious memories of their childhood physicians, the legends of Hippocrates and Maimonides, the discoveries of Pasteur and Fleming, and the clinical skills of Freud and Osler. Today's physician trust and respect have been earned, but largely by those who have gone before.

We, today's and tomorrow's physicians, must aspire to be like the best of our professional forebears. We must be hardworking, resourceful, and patient-centered. As Phillips and Haynes wrote (see chapter 8), we must "be there" when our patients need us. We must always act with integrity and do what is right for the patient, striving to be the physician our patients believe us to be.

Medicine's Future and Yours

Tomorrow's White Coat Tales

Some of the tales we will tell young physicians in the future will be about what happens today and tomorrow—perhaps in your examination room or hospital. Some of these stories will concern AIDS, which Oldstone calls "a plague as bad as any ever known" (p. 140). Other viruses also threaten us, including Ebola, Marburg, and Hanta viruses. Could one of them mutate in a way that matches or even exceeds the devastation caused by the 1918 influenza pandemic? Then there is the concern that avian influenza (H5N1) will become a pandemic with human-to-human transmission.

On the more positive side, we can expect many new developments in genetic screening and gene therapy. Electronic technology promises to revolutionize day-by-day patient care, with electronic medical records serving as the platform. In years to come, we will see innovations in messaging between patients and physicians, virtual office visits and home visits, online group therapy, and much more. Robotic surgery is already a reality, and we will see innovations that are difficult to imagine today. In the end, perhaps we will even begin to conquer some of America's actual causes of death, which include tobacco use, poor diet and physical inactivity, excessive alcohol consumption, motor vehicle accidents, careless sexual behavior, and illicit drug use (6).

Tomorrow and You

In the meantime, while the dramas that will generate tomorrow's tales are unfolding, what should you and I do? First of all, we should take good care of our families and ourselves and enjoy the practice of medicine—a rare privilege for which we should give thanks every day. Famed investor Warren Buffet has been quoted as saying, "When I go my office every morning, I feel like I'm going to the Sistine Chapel to paint" (7). My wish for you is that you share this feeling with Buffet and with me.

There is more. Medicine is much more than seeing your 20 patients in the office tomorrow, more than performing three operations or passing an endoscope four times in the morning, more than making hospital rounds or visiting a patient in the nursing home or whatever else your specialty calls for you to do in your workday. What is *more* is doing your part in regard to tomorrow's white coat tales.

How can you or I do this? How can we—in some small way—help pass on the history of medicine to the next generation? To accomplish this, I suggest five tasks:

- Enhance your personal knowledge about medicine's past. Begin a program of reading about medical giants, language, and culture. Choose among the books in the Bibliography or perhaps even Osler's reading list (see page 232). Become, in Osler's words, "close friends" with them. Keep an enrichment book at your bedside and read a little each night.
- Make the extra effort to learn about newly encountered medical terms and syndromes. Look up clinical word origins and search out the life stories of persons for whom diseases and syndromes are named. Then keep a notebook, entering new findings as you learn them.

- Become a medically oriented traveler. Use your personal tourism to expand your knowledge of medical history, visiting some of the sites listed above or by discovering some of your own. Involve your family in the exploration and learning.
- Add to the medical literature. You may find an intriguing connection between a current clinical finding and medical history. Perhaps you will have an insight involving a medical hero or one of the historic plagues. You may have noted a previously unreported cluster of diseases or an unusual manifestation of an illness. When you have a thought worth sharing, consider writing a short piece and submitting it for publication. If you do so, you have added a tale to medicine's anthology. Along the way, you will discover that writing for publication is a journey of education, self-discovery, and personal growth (8).
- Seek to develop a sense of how the medical information you use in daily practice has come not only from scientific "evidence-based" sources. Your medical knowledge and mine also has its roots in the lore of medicine. It began with the incense-burners, amulet-makers, and quasi-religious ritualists and evolved from those days through the centuries of discoveries to the knowledge we now take for granted. I urge you to stop often and reflect that every diagnostic maneuver, every therapeutic intervention, and every word and phrase in medicine come from some source, some person, or some event in history. The stories of these origins are medicine's *White Coat Tales*.

Thank you for reading my book. I will end, as I began 11 chapters ago, with a quote from Félix Martí-Ibáñez (p. 200):

In your future work, you will be in good company. The great physicians of history, the glorious figures of the past, will always be near you. When you perform a dissection, a red-bearded young man with flashing eyes, Andreas Vesalius, will be peering over your shoulder; when you conduct a physiological experiment, the melancholy, pensive eyes of William Harvey will be watching you; when you teach medicine, the venerable figure of William Osler with his Apollonian head will come and sit like a medical Goethe beside you; and when you approach the sickbed, the shades of Hippocrates, Sydenham, and Fleming will gather round to counsel you, the young princes [and princesses] of our profession.

References

1. Persian history: the National Museum of Medical Science. Available at: http://imp. lss.wisc.edu/~aoliai/historypage/thenationalmuseum.htm. Accessed May 18, 2007.
2. U.S. National Library of Medicine Web site. Available at: http://www.nlm.nih.gov. Accessed May 18, 2007.
3. Lipp MR. *Medical Landmarks USA: A Travel Guide to Historic Sites, Architectural Gems, Remarkable Museums and Libraries, and Other Places of Health-Related Interest.* New York, NY: McGraw-Hill; 1991.

4. Rojas-Burke J. Doctor and intervention outlast jeers and threats. *The Oregonian.* December 21, 2006:A1 and A10.
5. The Monster Drug. Available at: http://www.mendosa.com/monster.htm. Accessed May 18, 2007.
6. McGinnis JM, Foege WH. Actual causes of death in the United States. *JAMA.* 1993;270:2207–2212.
7. Klein M. *The Change Makers.* New York, NY: Henry Holt and Co.; 2003.
8. Taylor RB. *The Clinician's Guide to Medical Writing.* New York, NY: Springer; 2005.

Bibliography

Ackerknecht EH. *History and Geography of the Most Important Diseases.* New York, NY: Hafner; 1972.

Beighton P, Beighton G. *The Man Behind the Syndrome.* Heidelberg, Germany: Springer-Verlag, 1986.

Bloomfield RL, Chandler ET. *Pocket Mnemonics for Practitioners.* Winston-Salem, NC: Harbinger Medical Press; 1983.

Blumberg DR. *Whose What? Aaron's Beard to Zorna's Lemma.* New York, NY: Holt, Rinehart and Winston; 1969.

Bollet AJ. *Plagues and Poxes: The Impact of Human History on Epidemic Disease.* New York, NY: Demos; 2004.

Bordley J. *Two Centuries of American Medicine, 1776–1976.* Philadelphia, PA: Saunders; 1976.

Brallier JM. *Medical Wit and Wisdom.* Philadelphia, PA: Running Press; 1994.

Bryson B. *The Mother Tongue.* New York, NY: Perennial; 2001.

Cartwright FF. *Disease and History: The Influence of Disease in Shaping the Great Events of History.* New York, NY: Crowell; 1972.

Ciardi J. *A Browser's Dictionary and Native's Guide to the Unknown American Language.* New York, NY: Harper & Row; 1980.

Dirckx JH. *The Language of Medicine: Its Evolution, Structure, and Dynamics.* 2nd ed. New York, NY: Praeger; 1983.

Dorland's Illustrated Medical Dictionary. 30th ed. Philadelphia, PA: Saunders; 2003.

Durham RH. *Encyclopedia of Medical Syndromes.* New York, NY: Harper and Brothers; 1960.

Ellerin TB, Diaz LA Jr. Evidence-based medicine: 500 clues to diagnosis and treatment. Philadelphia: Lippincott, Williams and Wilkins; 2001.

Evans B, Evans C. *A Dictionary of Contemporary American Usage.* New York, NY: Random House; 1957.

Evans IH. *Brewer's Dictionary of Phrase and Fable.* New York, NY: Harper & Row; 1970.

Firkin BG, Whitworth JA. *Dictionary of Medical Eponyms.* Park Ridge, NJ: Parthenon; 1987.

Fortuine R. *The Words of Medicine: Sources, Meanings, and Delights.* Springfield, IL: Charles C. Thomas; 2001.

Fowler HW. *A Dictionary of Modern English Usage.* 2nd ed. New York, NY: Oxford University Press; 1965.

Garrison FH. *History of Medicine.* 4th ed. Philadelphia, PA: Saunders; 1929.

Gershen BJ. *Word Rounds.* Glen Echo, MD: Flower Valley Press; 2001.

Goodman LS, Gilman A. *The Pharmacological Basis of Therapeutics.* 5th ed. New York, NY: Macmillan, 1975.

Gould GM, Pyle WL. *Anomalies and Curiosities of Medicine.* New York, NY: Kessinger; 1956.

Haubrich WS. *Medical Meanings: A Glossary of Word Origins.* Philadelphia, PA: American College of Physicians; 1997.

Hendrickson R. *The Literary Life and Other Curiosities.* New York, NY: Viking; 1981.

Holt AH. *Phrase and Word Origins: A Study of Familiar Expressions.* New York, NY: Dover; 1961.

Huth EJ, Murray TJ. *Medicine in Quotations: View of Health and Disease Through the Ages.* Philadelphia, PA: American College of Physicians; 2006.

Inglis B. *A History of Medicine.* New York, NY: World; 1965.

Kennett F. *Folk Medicine Fact and Fiction.* New York, NY: Crescent Books; 1976.

Lambert EC. *Modern Medical Mistakes.* Bloomington, IN: Indiana University Press; 1978.

Magalini SI, Scrascia E. *Dictionary of Medical Syndromes.* 2nd ed. Philadelphia, PA: Lippincott; 1981.

Major RH. *Classic Descriptions of Disease.* 3rd ed. Springfield, IL: Charles C. Thomas; 1945.

Major RH. *Disease and Destiny.* New York, NY: Appleton-Century, 1936.

Maleska ET. *A Pleasure in Words.* New York, NY: Fireside Books; 1981.

Martí-Ibáñez F. *A Prelude to Medical History.* New York, NY: MD Publications, 1961.

Oldstone MBA. *Viruses, Plagues and History.* New York, NY: Oxford University Press; 1998.

Onions CT. *The Oxford Dictionary of English Etymology.* Oxford, UK: Clarendon Press; 1979.

Osler W. *Aequanimitas with Other Addresses to Medical Students, Nurses and Practitioners of Medicine.* 3rd ed. Philadelphia, PA: Blakiston; 1932.

Partridge E. *Origins: A Short Etymological Dictionary of Modern English.* New York, NY: Macmillan; 1979.

Pepper OHP. *Medical Etymology.* Philadelphia, PA: Saunders; 1949.

Porter R. *The Greatest Benefit to Mankind: A Medical History of Humanity.* New York, NY: Norton; 1997.

Rawson H. *A Dictionary of Euphemisms and Other Doubletalk.* New York, NY: Crown; 1981.

Reveno WS. *Medical Maxims.* Springfield, IL: Charles C. Thomas; 1951.

Sebastian A. *The Dictionary of the History of Medicine.* New York, NY: Parthenon; 1999.

Sherman IW. *The Power of Plagues.* Washington, DC: ASM Press, 2006.

Shipley JT. *Dictionary of Word Origins.* New York, NY: Philosophical Library; 1945.

Shryock RH. *Medicine and Society in America: 1660–1860.* Ithaca, NY: Cornell University Press; 1960.

Skinner HA. *The Origin of Medical Terms.* Baltimore, MD: Williams & Wilkins; 1949.

Strauss MB. *Familiar Medical Quotations.* Boston, MA: Little, Brown; 1968.

Train J. *Remarkable Words with Astonishing Origins.* New York, NY: Charles N. Potter; 1980.

Weekley E. *An Etymological Dictionary of Modern English.* New York, NY: Dover; 1967.

Weiss AB. *Medical Odysseys: The Different and Sometimes Unexpected Pathways to 20th Century Medical Discoveries.* New Brunswick, NJ: Rutgers University Press; 1991.

Index

Printed in the United States of America